BOSH!
HOW TO LIVE
VEGAN

SAVE THE PLANET AND
FEEL AMAZING

HENRY FIRTH & IAN THEASBY

wm

WILLIAM MORROW

An Imprint of HarperCollins*Publishers*

We'd like to dedicate this book to you. The very fact that you have this book in your hands is proof that you care greatly about the planet and all its inhabitants. It's people like you who are going to make a difference and, ultimately, change the world.

BOSH!
HOW TO LIVE
VEGAN

SAVE THE PLANET AND
FEEL AMAZING

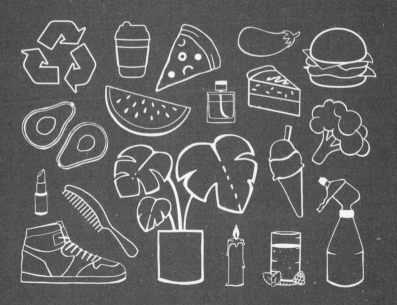

HENRY FIRTH & IAN THEASBY

CONTENTS

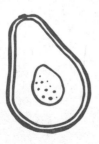
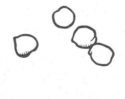

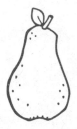

HOW?

(110)

A NOTE FROM HENRY

You'll have come to this book because you are ready to make a change. My journey to veganism started at a pretty tough time in my life.

At my lowest point, I was running a company that had raised millions of pounds, but I wasn't happy. My silicon dream had become a silicon nightmare. Around then, I took a trip to Japan to try to gain some clarity, and while I was there, I realized I needed to change my focus to make my mind healthy again. I rediscovered meditation, reading, exercise, and a work–life balance. On returning to the UK, I made the decision to act more responsibly with regard to my personal health and to find a meaningful purpose to my life. I wanted to use my skills to help the planet and, specifically, to help stop climate change in whatever way I could.

At the time, I was working with a close friend of mine, Ian. He went through all those dark times at work with me, and we not only worked together but also shared a house. Then one day he went vegan. I thought it was ridiculous. I made fun of him all the time. I was *that* guy. I had a freezer full of organic, free-range meat and a personal trainer that had me on a high-fat ketogenic diet. I wasn't going to eat Ian's dubious-looking curries.

Then I watched a documentary—*Cowspiracy*—that changed everything. I went vegan overnight. With the help of some friends, Ian and I set up our video channel, BOSH.TV, to show the world how to cook plant-based meals that meat eaters would love, and before long we'd had a billion views and were two-time *Sunday Times* bestselling authors.

Now we are regularly called upon to talk about vegan food on TV, radio, and at live events. And we love to share what we know and how we feel. But we think it's also important to recognize that we each have our own opinions, patterns, and issues.

To us, eating vegan food is the proverbial Band-Aid that we can personally stick on the broken planet to help it heal. But we know it's not that black and white. My dad was the first to let me know that flying to America a couple of times a year can generate as much carbon as being vegan can save. His choice to eat just a bit of meat every now and again, combined with his love of seasonal and locally grown vegetables and a lifestyle that involves very little air travel, is an environmentally friendly choice that works for him.

But however we look at it, the way most of us are eating now is not OK. The way we farm and make food is destroying the planet, the rainforests, and our health, and it is causing huge suffering for billions of animals.

The topic of food is a huge one—and our habits are all so ingrained in us around the world that it can be hard to imagine a different system from the one we currently live in. Yet, we are at a place in our history where we are lucky enough to be able to choose what we eat—in fact, there has never been so much choice! And with this choice comes the responsibility to make informed decisions.

We aren't preachy, holier-than-thou people, and this book won't be filled with propaganda and made-up facts. As sons of meat eaters, surrounded by meat eaters, who were brought up eating meat, we're going to show you why and how we went vegan. We're going to walk you through why we chose to live a vegan life, and why eating vegan, whether it's a few times a week or every day, could literally help you to save the planet, feel amazing, and live longer.

Whoever you are, wherever you are on your journey, we respect you, and we trust that you'll make your own informed decisions (even if they're different from ours) on how to live vegan.

A NOTE FROM IAN

As a vegan, I'm going to say something controversial: you can eat what you like.

Meat is what most people are brought up on. Eating it doesn't make you a bad person. And not eating meat, being veggie or vegan, doesn't make you a good person.

Henry and I remember the taste of meat well. We loved steak and roast dinners, and there's no question that burgers taste great. My mum is the daughter of a farmer. Our families and friends from home still eat meat and we still love them all dearly.

Our families definitely did not expect us to be running a vegan cooking channel, and they're always asking us why we went vegan. In this book is the answer to that. Mum, this book is for you!

We stopped eating animal products over four years ago. Since then we've built the biggest plant-based online video channel and written two bestselling cookbooks, showing people how to make delicious meals that taste even better than meat!

This book contains no propaganda. It's not designed to try and mess with your mind or turn you into clones of us. We've cited our sources and tried to avoid hyperbole. But there's no doubt, this *is* important.

If you're wondering why the number of vegans has more than quadrupled[1] in the past few years and why the number of flexitarians (people who are reducing the amount of meat they eat) is showing similar trends, then this book hopefully holds the answer.

If you're wondering why so many restaurants have added vegan choices or are shouting about their vegan offerings, then this book may explain why. Spoiler: the availability of vegan options is not down to an increasing number of vegans, it's down to an increasing number of meat reducers—those mindful meaties!

If you're wondering why Sir David Attenborough, or any news channel, declares we should reduce our meat and dairy intake to help the planet, then this book is for you. We'll share the background to this and give you practical advice on how you can make changes in your own life.

And, finally, if you're just interested in eating a few more vegan meals, either to help the planet, for your health, to save money, or because you're interested in trying some of the amazing new plant-based foods that are out there, then we'll help you do that, too. We'll show you how awesome vegan food can be for your mind, body, and soul.

All of this is aimed at you doing it your way. There is no one-size-fits-all solution.

Anyone who throws a black-and-white absolute answer at you—about anything—is misleading you. So, please come with us as we delve into the murky shades of gray, and we'll show you how the choice to eat vegan food, and to make vegan an ideal that we work toward, was the best decision we ever made. Ever.

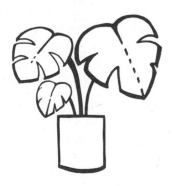

WHAT DOES VEGAN MEAN?

The Vegan Society's definition of veganism is living in a way that "seeks to exclude, as far as is possible and practicable, all forms of exploitation of, and cruelty to animals."

In fact, it was the founder of the Vegan Society who actually created the word "vegan." Based in the UK, the society supports vegans all over the world through information and campaigns, and registers products with its Vegan Trademark. We think the bit about it being "as far as is possible and practicable" is massively overlooked in most conversations about what it means to be vegan. Some people will tell you there are very strict rules about what you can and can't do if you want to be a "proper" vegan—but there aren't! When you start to really think about it deeply, it's nearly impossible to live 100% vegan. Animal products end up in the weirdest of places—from the ink in your printer, to the interior of your car, and even your money.

We see veganism as something to aim for. It's an ideal, a direction to move toward—we're still working on it, too—and however far you want to take it, that's OK with us. In this book, we want to show you the facts. You can use them however you want.

For some people being vegan is all about the food, while for others it's about other parts of their life, too, like their clothes or makeup, or the products they buy for their home. Maybe you just want to eat a few more plant-based meals each week, or swap your dairy milk and cheese for plant-based alternatives. That's amazing! What we've found is that even the small changes make a big difference. And not only to your life, but to those around you, too.

We started **BOSH!** three years ago, motivated to help the world eat more plants, as a means of reducing climate change. Our videos have reached millions of people, and we've lost count of the number who have gotten in touch to let us know that they've gone vegan, or eat far less meat, after trying one of our recipes. We are supportive of *whatever* positive action you take toward consuming fewer animal products and eating more plant-based foods. Maybe you've made a decision that all your main meals are going to be vegan, but you simply can't live without your nonvegan snacks—we're cool with that! Whether you go the whole hog (pun intended) or choose to start with a few smaller adjustments, it's about doing whatever is practical for *you*.

Before we went vegan, pretty much *every* meal we ate was built around something animal-based. At first, we admit, it was a bit of a challenge to go completely plant-based—Ian cooked *a lot* of brown curries in those early days . . . But things are much better now—there is so much choice out there! We are excited by the plant-based options on the supermarket shelves, the new vegan restaurants opening up every day, and the vegan options appearing on menus in even the most mainstream of fast-food outlets. And, of course, we've learned a huge amount along the way, too. We've learned how to cook really amazing vegan food, and we're so excited to be able to share that with you through our YouTube channel, Facebook, Instagram, and our books.

Our mission today remains the same as it was back then. We've all heard the facts. We all know about the increased risks of wildfires, extreme weather events, and rising sea levels. But recently, the language has changed. We are no longer talking about climate "change," but rather climate *crisis* and climate *emergency*. Hearing Sir David Attenborough, Greta Thunberg, and Professor Mike Berners-Lee talking on the BBC documentary *Climate Change—The Facts*, in clear and certain terms about the huge, extinction-level threats we face as a result of climate change, it brought everything even more keenly into focus for us. We watched, gripped in horror as the first climate refugees were forced from their homes by rising sea levels and at the deforestation spreading across the globe and the unprecedented California forest blazes in 2018. It's a lot, we know. And we don't want to depress or scare you.

But in the face of these terrifying events, it is easy to want to bury our heads in the sand and wait for the inevitable apocalypse. Thankfully, though, Sir David Attenborough, along with his copresenters, ended the show with perhaps their most important message of all: they finished by telling us what we can do about it.

The biggest way you can help our planet is to reduce your meat and dairy intake and move toward a more plant-based diet, become a flexitarian, go veggie, or go vegan.

There are so many ways to reduce your meat and dairy intake, but the most important thing of all is to make sure you do it your way.

You need to find a way to make plant-based eating work for you, in your life, right now. Perhaps a fully plant-based, vegan diet is just too big a change at the moment. If so, then a few simple adjustments to your usual routine can still deliver some amazing improvements. Even switching out beef in your diet and moving toward more sustainable options is a really powerful change. Or maybe you want to play with being a flexitarian before you take the plunge—eating mainly plant-based but with the occasional meat, fish, and dairy.

Beyond Meat, the groundbreaking new vegan burger company, says 93% of their sales are from meat eaters,[2] showing that the interest in everyone eating less meat is most definitely on the rise. This means that the buying power of flexitarians is causing a huge spike in sales of vegan products! Being vegan is actually being made easier by people becoming flexitarian, because it increases the demand for quality and easy-to-find nonanimal products. So even eating a few more plant-based meals will make a big difference in our overall global consumption.

You don't have to be a full-blown card-carrying vegan. You don't have to wear socks and sandals or put hemp seeds in your smoothies. It is not about that. It's about *reducing* your meat and dairy intake, whatever that means for you.

Think about what has brought you to this point. Why do you want to live vegan? Is it due to the environment, your health, the animals, or for humanitarian reasons? Are you planning to change the way that you shop for nonfood products as well? Some clothes, personal care products, and makeup are made from animal products—do you plan to cut those out? Or just focus on food for now? Considering all your options will help you stay committed to your decision. It's a really good time to think about your life and what you plan to do, then make daily decisions keeping you in line with those aims.

It's simple. Choose animal-free products. *As far as is right for you.*

As consumers, our biggest power is in what we buy. Reducing the amount of money we spend on animal agriculture is the single best way we can, as consumers, start to make a positive impact. We're going to show you how to vote against the meat, dairy, and animal products in your life, without compromising choice, flavor, or lifestyle. You'll see how easy it is, you'll feel better and healthier, and you'll know that you are drastically reducing your carbon footprint, too.

We'll help you **BOSH!** your kitchen, your bathroom, and your life. We'll show you how to remove animal products and turn your fave meaty meals plant-based. We'll give you all the tools you need so you can save the planet and feel amazing.

In Great Britain, the number of vegans quadrupled between 2014 and 2018. There were about 600,000 vegans in 2018, or 1.16% of the population.[3] During that time, **BOSH!** launched, making recipes for our books and our channels, where our videos have been viewed 1.5 billion times. That's a lot of views!

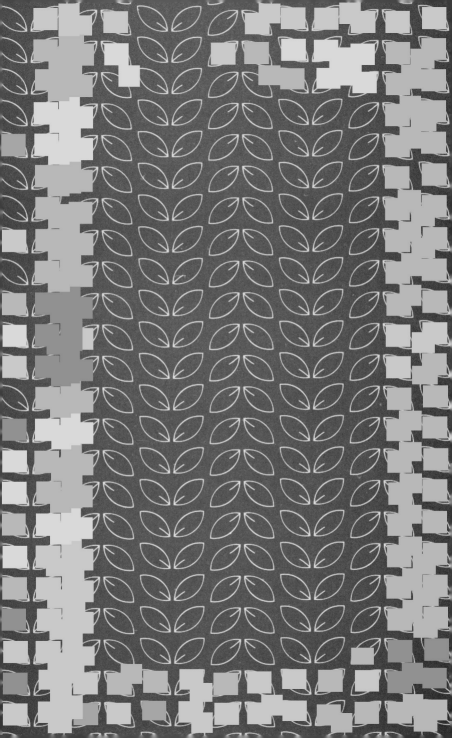

WHY?

1

SAVE
THE
PLANET

We all want to make a positive change for the world, but before we show you how you can do that, we think it's important to understand exactly why veganism is a part of that change.

We'll give you a heads-up now that it can make tough reading at times, but we can't shy away from the facts and so in this section we're going to start with a few home-hitting truths. They were a real wake-up call for us, and they help keep us motivated every day to do what we do.

About one-quarter of our personal carbon footprint in the UK is down to the food and drink we consume.

JOSEPH POORE

Researcher at the School of Geography and the Environment, the University of Oxford.

As individuals, the single biggest and most important thing we can do to reduce climate change is to cut down our meat and dairy intake . . .

And the science on this is absolutely clear-cut.

PROFESSOR MIKE BERNERS-LEE
in *Climate Change—The Facts*

Pow. What a great milestone!
Now we are all talking about meat
and dairy as being a huge part of
the problem, we can go about
starting to fix it.

It's sadly undeniable that our addiction to steaks, hamburgers,
and cheese is a core part of the problem. It's pretty clear
to us that we need to reduce our intake of those so we can
reduce the amount of greenhouse gases we are releasing
into the atmosphere. As individuals, that's the most powerful
thing we can do to reduce our carbon footprint.

There have been five mass extinctions in the history of our
planet. This period that we are living in now has been termed
the "sixth mass extinction."[4] This is an entirely human-
caused extinction. We've killed half of all wildlife in the last
40 years,[5] and since the rise of human civilization, 83% of
wild mammals have been lost.[6] We're causing the biggest
extinction since the dinosaurs, and the first extinction where
the cause—us—is acting through choice.

What has brought this about? Well, the loss of animals is partly
due to human overpopulation, but also overconsumption.
There are a lot of us on this little planet, yes, but our repeated
acts of killing for food and destroying habitats are the main

destroyers of wildlife.[7] Humans have modified more than half of the Earth's surface according to their own aims,[8] and it is estimated that 26% of the entire Earth's surface is now used for livestock grazing.[9]

It's not just wildlife that's at risk either. Perhaps the bigger, more frightening danger that we are currently facing is the warming of the planet. Scientists have warned that the "catastrophic" level of 35°F warming is a nightmare we need to avoid,[10] and while this has been popularly framed as a doomsday-like worst-case scenario, in practice, that catastrophic 35°F warming is more like the best-case scenario.[11]

Increased levels of greenhouse gases, including methane and carbon dioxide, are trapping more heat in the Earth's atmosphere. This prevents it from cooling down properly, and as a result the planet is warming up rapidly, in turn causing dramatic melting of the ice caps and an increasing number of climate-related disasters.[12]

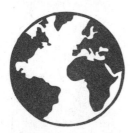

Carbon levels in the atmosphere are at their highest in 650,000 years. [13]

A warming planet also means we can expect more global conflicts.[14] We were surprised by this at first, but it is inevitable: as the natural resources people depend on—water, food, fuel, etc.—become increasingly limited, and unpredictable weather events cause climatic damage to landscapes and communities, governments will find it harder to protect and manage their societies. Severe droughts,[15] drowned coastal cities,[16] and millions of climate migrants from scorched, desertified countries[17] will leave people feeling uncertain about their futures, resulting in widespread instability and political unrest.

These threats will materialize for the world's poorest first,[18] particularly those around the equator, and there are already communities whose homes are being threatened or destroyed by climate activity across Africa, Asia, South America, and even Alaska,[19] where temperatures are rising more dramatically than elsewhere. Meanwhile, our overconsumption is also affecting the poorest. Isn't it terrifying to learn that although we produce enough food to feed every human on the planet, over 800 million people go to bed hungry each day?[20]

When we learnt these facts, we have to admit that we found ourselves losing faith in humanity for a while. As soon as you hear statistics like these, it's easy to feel resigned and deflated—as though you don't have any control. But we pulled ourselves back out of that hole and realized that there is something we can do—we can all act in a way that does some good for the world. Let's use these depressing and humbling facts as a motivator to make a change!

We know we are lucky to live in the Western world. A world where we import avocados from the other side of the globe to take photos of them in our meals and show people on the internet. It's not useful for anyone to go around feeling endlessly guilty every day about all that we have, but we do need to acknowledge how privileged we are.

We may not have intentionally caused these problems, but indirectly, by just existing and enjoying the modern world we live in—with all its luxuries and technologies—we have. We must take some responsibility.

We are young professionals who travel on a regular basis around the UK and also around the world. We buy and eat food when we're out and about. We enjoy our laptops, our phones—in fact, our whole living stems from being online 24/7. We buy clothes that are in fashion and we don't refuse napkins or take our lunch in a metal box every day.

We have to own up and accept some responsibility for our choices.

Human civilization has been around for about 12,000 years. The addition of excess carbon dioxide and other greenhouse gases into the planet's atmosphere has all happened in our lifetime, in the last 30 years.[21, 22] And science shows us we have about the same amount of time left to fix it.[23]

It's like some kind of sci-fi film plot in which the entire history of humanity as we know it lies in the hands of just two generations. And at this point in the story, it doesn't look much like a happy ending.

How terrifying is that?! But also, how *amazing* that it is potentially still possible to fix it.

There is, in fact, a lot to be positive about. As we all become more aware of what needs to be done, it's incredibly encouraging to see people all around the world taking action and making great strides in the name of climate change and the environment.

The scientific
evidence is that if
we have not taken
dramatic action
within the next
decade, we could face
irreversible damage
to the natural world
and the collapse of
our societies.[24]

SIR DAVID ATTENBOROUGH

ANIMAL WELFARE

Climate change isn't the only reason people come to veganism. There are three main motivations that lead people toward wanting to adopt a more plant-based way of eating and living:

1. The environment
2. The treatment of animals
3. Health

Whatever the reason you started out on your vegan journey, it's inevitable that the more you read around the subject, the more you will start to care about the other two reasons as well.

Ian started eating vegan as part of a health kick one January, but then it quickly became more about animal welfare and the environment, too. Henry came at it with climate change as his main motivation, but then found a renewed love of animals, and enjoyed better health to boot.

If you are fully engaged in your vegan journey—which we encourage you to be at all times—it's impossible not to start caring about the cruelty inflicted on animals as part of current farming practices around the world—from animals packed into small living spaces or separating mothers from their children in the dairy industry, to the catastrophic destruction of wild fish populations from commercial fishing.

We're often asked what's so wrong about organic, free-range meat sourced from herds that roam freely across acres of beautiful fields and whose farmer talks to them every day and knows them all by name. Surely that's OK, right?

Well, aside from the debate over whether it's ever OK to kill another creature, the main issue we have here is that it's simply not sustainable for everyone on the planet to eat in this way. Most people don't eat, don't have access to, or simply can't afford to eat meat that has been raised in this way. And we simply don't have the space on the planet to do it either. Many animal products on supermarket shelves come from animals that have been raised in poor conditions in factory farms, farmed cheaply to meet with demand.[25, 26]

We want to move toward food and lifestyle choices that work for everyone, not a select few.

HEALTH

The majority of people choosing to eat more plants are actually doing so for health reasons.[27] Although animal welfare is a very close second.

We know, firsthand, how amazing eating a vegan diet can make you feel. Almost instantly we both felt lighter—we lost weight, sure, but we also felt lighter in ourselves, too. We slept better, our digestion was better, our hair was thicker—and a surprising benefit was that our hangovers were easier, too! Result! (Although it did take us a while to find the perfect vegan alternative to a hangover bacon sandwich . . . To be honest, that was one of the main motivations behind our Big Breakfast Bagel in our second book, **BISH BASH BOSH!**) We also found our energy levels were easier to sustain, rather than having a drop in energy or evening slump in front of the TV.

That's not to say all vegan food is healthy—you can easily be unhealthy on a vegan diet, as you can on any diet. But generally, if you're eating more veg, then you're going to quickly see improvements in how you look and feel.

As a happy side effect, too, we found we became more conscious of everything we were putting into our bodies. Reading the backs of labels to see if they were vegan or not (more on this later) meant we also became more aware of other ingredients we might want to avoid—the additives and preservatives and colorings that we all know aren't doing us any good. Of course, we sometimes choose things that we know aren't very healthy—it's all about balance after all, and we both have a MASSIVE sweet tooth!—but we're now a bit more aware of our choices.

But don't just take our word for it; there's plenty of science to back it up, too.

A diet rich in fruit and veg is higher in vitamins, nutrients, and fiber. And since it's much harder to overeat if you're mainly eating veg, it's harder to gain a lot of excess weight. In fact, a growing body of doctors, dieticians, and athletes now say that a plant-based diet is the best way to fuel and protect our bodies. There is increasing evidence that eating a well-planned plant-based diet is linked with lower body weight,[28] lower rates of obesity,[29] diabetes,[30] and heart disease.[31] For more on why you'll feel AMAZING on a plant-based diet, see page 66.

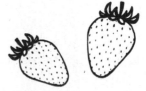

SO WHAT CAN WE DO ABOUT IT?

Climate change is a complicated problem (err . . . understatement!) with lots of different perspectives to consider. There are so many contributing factors to climate change that there's no one clear way out of the mess. When you're faced with such a multitude of facts and figures, arguments and opinions, we know how easy it can be to feel analysis paralysis! We're so overwhelmed by the complexity of the problem, we never decide how best to tackle it. Perhaps that's why historically, as a global community, we've not done an awful lot about it so far.

Leading bodies say we need to embark on a World War II–level effort to combat climate change,[32] and yet it's definitely a more abstract problem to come to grips with—harder to picture, harder to explain, harder to solve. This can leave us frozen in indecision, right down to the smallest of everyday choices. There are so many people with different answers to the problem that it's hard to know what to believe. We're blocked by confusion and doubt.

Are plastic straws to blame? Should we all buy electric cars? Stop taking flights and start going on vacation by train? Where does food waste fit into the problem? Do we have to go veggie? But surely eating local meat and eggs is better than eating avocados and quinoa from South America?

On a personal level, the main barrier we think we all face is a feeling of helplessness.

What can we really achieve as individuals? How can we change what's being done by billions of people, if even governments and big businesses are not able to stop it? While some people are unwilling to make changes to help the greater good, surely the vast majority of humanity would want to help, if only they knew how?

Ian went through a phase of using bamboo toothbrushes and tried to live as close to zero waste as he could. But in our job—developing recipes every day—it's almost impossible to live like this. We made a decision that we could have more impact if we concentrated on our main message of making delicious plant-based food available to everyone. We use sustainable ingredients as much as we can, but we can't do everything all at the same time. And that's OK—we do what we can.

We held our love for steak and roast dinners on a proverbial weighing scale and compared it with our love for the world and the future we wanted for the next generation. We loved food, had our favorite meals, and didn't want to give them up. Henry's obsession with fish and chips, swimming in tartar sauce, held him back for a while. But as we looked deeper into the facts, we were unable to resist the reality of the situation.

THE MAIN CAUSES OF CLIMATE CHANGE

There are two main causes of climate change that far outweigh any others: transport and animal agriculture.

Let's start with transport. A flight from London to New York costs the Arctic 32 square feet of ice per person.[33] One thing we can all do to reduce our carbon footprint is to consider flying less and avoiding air-freighted goods. Following the rule of supply and demand, if we fly less, fewer flights will take place and air travel will cause fewer carbon dioxide emissions in the future. The same goes for choosing to drive electric cars instead of standard diesel or gasoline vehicles.

Animal agriculture, however, has much farther reaching consequences. Cutting down your transport emissions reduces your greenhouse gas output. This is a simple equation.

A vegan diet is probably the single biggest way to reduce your impact on planet Earth. Not just greenhouse gases, but global acidification, eutrophication, land use, and water use. It is far bigger than cutting down on your flights or buying an electric car.[34]

JOSEPH POORE
Researcher at the School of Geography and the Environment, the University of Oxford

Using the same rule of supply and demand, cutting down on animal products reduces carbon dioxide and methane emissions, land and water use, rainforest deforestation, and destruction of wildlife.

If going vegan seems a stretch too far, then even just eating one more plant-based meal per week is a powerful action. If everyone in the UK dropped meat from one meal a week, we could slash emissions by more than 8%, equivalent to taking 16 million cars off the road. It would also mean a 23% reduction in the UK's domestic and international farmland use and a 2% reduction in our water use.[35] And in the US, if everyone replaced chicken with plant-based foods in one meal per week, the carbon dioxide savings would be equivalent to taking half a million cars off the roads.[36]

The international committee for climate change has said that in order for the UK to reach their emissions targets of a net zero emissions economy by 2050, households will need to undergo at least a 20% reduction in their beef, lamb, and dairy consumption.

Source: *Climate Change—The Facts*

So the science really is that clear. The single biggest thing we can all do as individuals, much bigger than changing our approach to transport, is to eat more vegan, more plant-based meals. Given the wealth of experts across all fields of research telling us to eat fewer animal products, it's time to act. We now know we can fight climate change with diet change. We are now aware of the consequences of our actions. Past this point, *we're* to blame if we don't take action.

Will we rise to the challenge and save the world we live in, for ourselves and future generations? Our preferences for meat and dairy have led us to destroy the planet, turning forest and grasslands into grazing lands because we love the taste of hamburgers. Come on, guys! That's madness!

We make enough food to feed everyone on the planet, and yet nearly a billion people starve. We feed the food that they could eat to cattle so that we can eat steak. Eighty-two percent of the world's starving children live in countries where food is fed to animals, which are then killed for meat and exported—eaten by wealthier individuals in developed countries like the US, UK, and mainland Europe.[37]

It's time we stepped up to the (vegan) plate and took some positive action.

Animal farming uses up **83%** of global agricultural land, but provides just **18%** of global calories. [38]

These were the facts that we faced four years ago that led us, as extremely devoted lifelong meat eaters, to make the decision we made. We loved the taste of meat and dairy, but that didn't sit right with us. We wanted to make a change. So we went vegan.

That's all the bad news out of the way. Now for the good news.

Making the decision to cut animal products out of our diet was the best decision we ever made. It's not restrictive. We eat a wonderful variety of foods and have all the flavors and choices we want.

Since becoming vegan we've both become infinitely more open-minded about our food choices. Closing the door on meat, dairy, and fish has enabled us to open up a thousand other exciting plant-based doors. Our attitude to food now is far more broad-minded than ever before and, as a direct result, our diet is more diverse than we would ever have imagined.

Nothing will benefit
human health and
increase the chances
for survival of life
on Earth as much
as the evolution to a
vegetarian diet.

ALBERT EINSTEIN

Ian especially really enjoys "veganizing" dishes, and cooking delicious vegan food has become our hobby and passion and our job. When we nail a brand-new dish, and we mean really nail it, we get a dizzy sense of satisfaction. High-fives, fist-pumps, and whoops are all commonplace in our kitchen. One of the dishes we're most proud of is our Crispy Chili Tofu, which mimics one of Henry's old prevegan favorites, Crispy Chili Beef, perfectly.

Contrary to what the media would have us believe, choosing to become vegan is a powerful and motivating change and it is actually really easy to do. The power to save the planet is literally in your hands.

Taking shorter showers or using your bathwater to flush the toilet will all have a great impact. Replacing your toothbrush with a wooden one and cycling everywhere will help in so many ways, too. But avoiding meat and dairy is the single biggest way to reduce your impact on the Earth. A plant-based diet—or a more plant-based diet—is better for the planet and will drastically reduce your annual carbon footprint.

Even the least sustainable plant-based food is more sustainable than the most sustainable animal products. [39] That's something we like to remind ourselves if we ever worry about using ingredients that have questionable sustainability or have traveled far.

Just eat more plants.

A global switch to more veggie-focused diets could reduce greenhouse gas emissions by **two-thirds** and save **8 million lives** by 2050.[40]

Red meat is responsible for **10 to 40 times** as many greenhouse gas emissions as veggies and grains.[41] Beef creates up to **231 lb** of greenhouse gases **per 3.5 oz** of meat, compared to tofu, which produces less than **7.8 lb**.[42]

Put simply, cows create a lot of methane—basically they fart and burp a lot. Feeding cows grass is a very powerful way to create greenhouse gases. And dairy is not off the hook either. It takes about 264 gallons of water to make 1 quart of dairy milk, compared to 78 gallons for the same amount of soy milk.[43] The least sustainable plant-based milk is significantly more sustainable, from the perspective of emissions, land use, and carbon footprint, than the most sustainable dairy milk.[44]

It's also worth noting that by supporting dairy production, you are still supporting meat production.

Meat and dairy are part of the same manufacturing process, subject to the same questionable welfare issues, and retired dairy cows are often used for meat. It's not much of a life . . .

People love dairy though. Cold milk on cereal, melted cheese on toast, clotted cream on scones, milk chocolate, whey protein, lattes . . . the list goes on and on. For a lot of people, dairy's a difficult thing to kick because it's everywhere. A couple of hours spent reading blog posts and watching videos that highlight the problems that surround the dairy industry in terms of ethics, health, and the environment should show you that dairy isn't all that cool.

Dairy alternatives have really improved over the past couple of years, and as they get more popular, which they will, the products available are only going to get even better, making the transition away from dairy much easier. See pages 140–141 for more on the plant-based alternatives that we enjoy regularly.

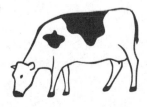

SO HOW EXACTLY DOES EATING VEGAN HELP?

All the energy we ingest through food comes originally from plants. This is the energy cycle we learned about in school. We are able to harvest and eat those plants to get all the energy, nutrients, minerals, and vitamins we need from them (more on this later).

When we rear animals for eating, we take this efficient form of plant energy and use it to sustain animals, like cows and sheep, so we can eat them later. This is much less efficient! Also, since animals are living creatures, most of their food is actually used for energy for their own day-to-day activity. Only a tiny fraction of the nutrients and energy in the food they eat ends up in the meat we buy. Cows convert only 4% of the proteins and 3% of the calories of the plants we feed them into beef[45]—97% of the calories they consume is completely lost to us. To produce 2.25 lb of beef requires over 3,434 gallons of water, a water footprint six times larger than for beans.[46] Meat accounts for 22% of all water use.[47]

According to researcher Joseph Poore, from Oxford University, about 55% of the world's land is farmed, and 80–85% of this is used to raise animals. [48] If as much of the land currently set aside for grazing animals regrows as trees, it will help remove carbon from the atmosphere—it is estimated there could be a reduction in greenhouse gases by as much as 30–50%. In addition, more than a billion extra tons of food crops could go to humans if we stopped feeding them to animals.[49]

So not only is a plant-based diet better for the planet in terms of the processes involved in rearing animals, but it can free up land for animals to live naturally again, and trees can grow in those spaces, which can then start to reduce the amount of carbon in the atmosphere. This is still the best approach for getting carbon out of the atmosphere—known as rewilding. It involves restoring natural forests, mangroves, salt marshes, and seagrass beds. These natural habitats are the best way researchers have identified of removing carbon dioxide from the atmosphere. And it would solve both climate breakdown and the extinction of species at the same time.[50]

Of course, we're not suggesting it's as simple as everyone, worldwide, stopping eating meat and redistributing the grain intended for animals to feed hungry people while we all start planting trees. At the global level we need to consider the complexities of politics, the mechanisms of food distribution, and the realities of farmers' livelihoods. And at the local level we need to consider things like soil health, crop cycling, and animal habitats.

We're not claiming there's some kind of magic solution, but the answer lies in this direction. These facts go to show how inefficient our current main choice of protein is, and why it's literally chewing up the Earth's resources.

WHAT ABOUT THE FARMER?

A note from Ian

I grew up in a reasonably big city. I love cities. I like their vibrancy, the people, the history, the architecture, and the energy. Having said this, I also love the countryside. I was lucky enough to spend a good chunk of my childhood in a small (and I mean very small) village called Gunthorpe.

My grandparents Charlie and Winnie owned and ran a small arable farm there. I have many fond memories of that farm. The memories mostly revolve around my grandma's wonderful cooking, but also exploring the old farm buildings and riding around in my grandad's tractor as he ploughed fields, planted seeds, and harvested crops.

I look back now, and realize that my grandfather worked bloody hard. All farmers do. When I say "worked bloody hard" I don't mean, "I got to the office at 9 a.m., hammered out some emails, then had lunch, had a meeting, smashed out a couple of spreadsheets, and was home at 6:30 p.m." I mean, "I woke up at 4:30 a.m., headed to one of my huge fields, smashed out some back-breaking labor until it got too dark to carry on, got home at 10 p.m., went to bed, and hit repeat the next day. Every day."

I understand how hard farmers work and I've got nothing but the utmost respect for their tremendous work ethic. However, having said that, I wholeheartedly believe that some of the practices used in farming need to be reevaluated and reformed. As the UK edges ever closer toward a more vegan way of life, and demand for vegan products grows and demand for nonvegan products declines, it's absolutely essential we give our farmers the tools, education, and incentives they need to adapt and thrive. We need to work with farmers to harness their unquestionable and inspiring work ethic and experience, and include them as a big, important part of the inevitable switch to plant-based living.

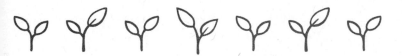

We've been talking a lot about meat, but we shouldn't ignore our sea-dwelling friends either.

Half of all marine life has been lost in the last **40 years**[51] and **87%** of fish populations are fully or over-exploited.[52]

We've already killed **90%** of big ocean predatory fish,[53] and it's been predicted that our world will **run out** of saltwater fish by **2048**.[54]

Increasing sea temperatures have destroyed coral reefs and all coral reefs are projected to be **lost by 2050**.[55]

Fishing is also a grossly inefficient way of eating; for every **1 lb** of fish caught, up to **5 lb** of unintended marine species are caught and discarded as by-kill.[56]

FEEDING A GROWING POPULATION

There's another thing to consider when thinking about the sustainability of our current diets. Our nutritional needs are going to evolve over the next few decades with the human population expected to reach more than 9 billion by 2050— a third higher than it is today.[57]

So what's the answer? Meat? No. Increasing annual meat production is a bad idea, however we do it. All approaches will use more land, create more deforestation, more climate change, more loss of biodiversity.[58] Feeding grain to livestock increases demand for grain and drives up prices, making it harder for the world's poor to feed themselves. If all grain were fed to humans, we could feed an extra 3.5 billion people.[59]

As Oxford University's Joseph Poore explains, fossil fuels represent about **61%** of today's emissions.

Some estimates say as much as **40%** of historic global warming is caused by forest clearance that was undertaken to make way for animal agriculture.

Currently, **25,000** species are threatened with extinction because of agriculture. Freeing up the land given over to animal farming will take some of this pressure off the global biodiversity crisis.

It will also reduce our nitrogen and phosphorus pollution, and will reduce acid rain by about **a third**.

A plant-based diet will reduce the amount of water we need to produce our food by **25%**.[60]

Yes, there are exciting developments in lab-grown meats and these could herald cheaper, less cruel forms of meat production. Many people are also big advocates of insect protein, although the morality of farming and killing gazillions of insects is still not in line with our moral standpoint. And both are still mildly processed, lab-made foodstuffs.

What about soy then? Soy is a great source of protein for those on a plant-based diet, although it is also the main cause of rainforest deforestation, which is being torn down to provide land to support it. This is an argument often used by antivegans, but let's remember that while around 70% of the world's soy is fed directly to livestock, only 6% is turned into human food.[61] (See page 54 for more on soy.)

In short, moving to a more plant-based diet is better for the planet and will reduce emissions. It will free up more land, which can then be rewilded and start to draw down carbon and solve our biodiversity crisis. And all the grain and soy that is currently fed to animals can be used to help feed the poorest nations. And the water that is not used for rearing those animals can be used for irrigating crops.

Of course, we appreciate that it is all far more complicated than that. There are good farms and bad farms. And conditions and practices differ all across the world. We all know people who keep chickens as egg-laying pets, and we can't really compare them with a 1,000-strong battery farm where chickens never see the light of day.

There are bad ways to farm vegetables, too, and we're not advocating a move to more monocrops.

However, ultimately, wherever your meat, fish, or dairy is coming from, it is a less environmentally friendly choice than any plant-based food.

A plant-based meal is more sustainable than one containing animal products. And so, the more plants you eat, the better.

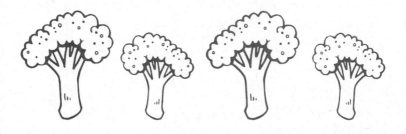

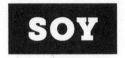

IS IT BAD FOR ME, AND IS IT BAD FOR THE PLANET?

Depending on who you are, you might see soy as either a wonderful health food or a risky ingredient to be avoided. And as far as the planet is concerned, there are differing opinions about how soy for humans is affecting the health of the planet. Some see it as the cure-all for our planet's woes, and some see it as the cause of rainforest deforestation. Let's delve into them both.

Soy is, on balance, a health food.

Some people, as part of some research from the '90s, formed the opinion that soy could be bad for your hormonal health. They drew inferences from the fact that soy contains estrogen-like compounds and speculated that it could mess with the hormonal balance of both women and men in different ways. These studies have largely been disproven now, and recent research shows that moderate consumption of soy foods can actually have some benefits.[62] Even a correlational relationship is not maintained, so largely we know this is not the case.

On the other hand, soy is a very powerful and healthful plant-based protein. It's a complete protein, containing all the nine essential amino acids we need in our diets (see page 150 for more on these). And it's a good source of omega-3 fats, iron, zinc, and calcium.

Soy fields are a cause of rainforest deforestation, but this soy is grown for animal feed.

Significant amounts of the Amazon rainforest are being destroyed every day, and these trees are crucial to our planet's survival. They are the lungs of our planet, and their loss is a significant factor in contributing to climate change.

A large amount of the rainforest deforestation occurs to make way for large, monocrop soy fields. This has been used regularly to illustrate that vegans" choice of soy milk is poor. But that's not the full story!

Eighty percent of the soy that is grown in the Amazon (the soy for which the rainforests are being destroyed) is fed to animals,[63] and indeed up to 90% of the rainforest's total deforestation is for animal agriculture.[64] But as we've seen, only 6% of the soy produced globally is consumed by humans.[65] So, while it is true that the megafields of soy are causing mass destruction of the rainforest, it's the animal agriculture industry that is causing it and utilizing the soy.

Also, when comparing the environmental impact that soy has on the planet versus an animal-based protein like beef, you should take into consideration all the soy the animal has consumed as part of its lifecycle. When framed like this it seems silly to compare the two. Rearing an animal is a much less efficient way to get protein, with only a fraction of the energy that is fed to the animal as plants being available to humans as meat. (See page 46.)

So, despite what many people would have you believe, you should feel free to consume soy with a clear conscience, from both a health and environmental perspective. It's good for your body and is much more environmentally friendly, when you look at all the factors involved, than eating a comparable animal protein. Miso, soy sauce, soy milk, edamame, tofu, and tempeh are all wonderful choices for you to include in your diet. We highly recommend getting on board with soy. It doesn't deserve its bad reputation, and in fact is part of the solution to the planet's ills, not part of the problem.

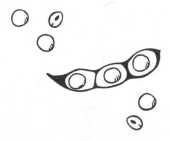

We can literally save the world by eating more plants.

CAN I REALLY MAKE A DIFFERENCE?

When we told our friend Naushard we'd gone vegan, he exclaimed that he'd found a flaw in our plan. He discovered that the motivation was climate change. And so, with a devilish look in his eye, he told us jokingly (or not jokingly) that for every steak we didn't eat, he was going to eat two steaks!

Great banter. Naushard is a funny guy. But let's delve into his threat for a moment. Not only did he not buy into our logic about cutting out meat having a positive impact, he didn't think that our not eating meat was going to make any difference at all. But he was also threatening to ensure that our change didn't make any tangible difference anyway, by upping his meat intake to counter our meat decrease. Funny. And kind of evil.

The last time we saw Naushard, we were shocked to hear that he had given up meat. "I don't eat steak anymore. I'm still eating fish, but no more steaks."

To hear him backtrack was a genuine shock. He is the last person you would expect to go back on his word. He would prefer to keep the joke going at the expense of the truth if it made it funnier. And here he was admitting that he had not only broken his promise, but had done a total about-face and joined us in the beef-free camp!

We see this all the time. We love it and it's one of the best things about our job. Talk to any vegan, and they'll have a story like this one. And it goes to show that you really *do* make a difference to those around you. We all affect everyone we come into contact with. What we are saying is that the system will never change if you don't change first. Often, too, we've found it's the ones who mock you the most who join you in the end—just like Henry used to laugh at Ian when he first went vegan!

Every big change in history has been started by a small collection of individuals, striving for a better world.

Whether it's the creation of the United Nations as a peacekeeping organization after World War II,[66] the abolition of slavery, or the global, ongoing move away from tobacco, these movements toward a better world were spearheaded by individuals changing their own views and actions, which in turn affected the views of others.

One person can make a difference to those around them. And slowly those people make a difference to those around them. The best way to make a change is to start with yourself. Change yourself first—since that's the thing you can control.

When people ask us why we're vegan, one of our responses is: "To avoid awkward conversations with our unborn children." Our generation—and the generation before us—has presided over the biggest extinction event in recent history, and it is the next generation that will pay the price for our inaction.

You really can make a difference to the world just by virtue of the decisions you make.

There can be no greater way to care for the happiness of others than to preserve the planet and future for them. The predictions of where the planet may end up otherwise are too grave to consider. We owe it to our young people to do something about climate change before it's too late. The effects of our actions will be felt by them. They will be clearing up our mess. Think about the conversations you'll have with them in the future. "What did you do when we could have stopped climate change, Daddy?!"

It may feel easier to avoid responsibility by thinking that the problem is bigger than us, or has been around longer than us. But to put it into perspective, consider how long humans have existed, and how recently climate change has escalated.

Humans have been on the planet for 12,000 years, but it's only in the past 140 years that we"ve burned fossil fuels, which has caused a lot of our current problems. Just 30 years ago, we knew most of what we know now about climate change, and we nearly put the wheels in motion to stop it. But we didn't. And since then we have done almost everything in our power to make it worse. We have a couple of decades to stop complete, irreversible disaster. It's crunch time.[67]

We can't sit back and do nothing. Let's spend our time on Earth trying to fix what we've broken—and enjoy some amazing food along the way!

YOUR MONEY IS YOUR VOTE

The money you spend is a vote for how you believe the world should be. Every single thing you buy fuels the economy. Every plant-based product that you buy tells the global economy that you want more plant-based—and therefore more sustainable—products. And every animal product that you buy tells the global economy that you want to continue to consume animal products, which are, we know, significantly worse for the planet.

What the world needs, for us to survive, is for us to spend our money on delivering change. If enough of us change our buying habits, then we can take our planet off the pressure cooker. We can start to put measures in place to cool it again, while letting the animal kingdom recover.

NOW IT'S YOUR TURN

Right now, let's take a moment to think about how we can all make a few simple changes to what we buy to help make a real difference.

- What do you spend your money on?

- What is the money that you spend demanding from our economy?

- Are there any changes that you could make to start persuading food producers to act more sustainably?

- If you do eat meat, how often?

- Do you think you could reduce it?

66

What happens next is up to us all. We now stand at a unique point in our planet's history, one where we must all share responsibility both for our present well-being and for the future of life on Earth.

Every one of us has the power to make changes and make them now. Our wonderful natural world and the lives of our children and grandchildren and all those who follow them, depend upon us doing so.

SIR DAVID ATTENBOROUGH
Climate Change—The Facts

GRETA THUNBERG

In 2018, at the age of just 15, Swedish schoolgirl Greta Thunberg protested outside government buildings about the need to take action on climate change. She caught the attention of the media, and went on to inspire hundreds of thousands of students in countries all around the world to follow her action with "school strikes for climate." In March 2019 an estimated 1.4 million students from 112 countries joined her in strikes and protests. And another global strike in May 2019 saw 125 countries getting involved. Greta's passion for her cause led to a nomination for the Nobel Peace Prize. So powerful and far-reaching has her influence been that it is known by some as the "Greta Thunberg effect."

Greta has since staged a TEDx Talk, spoken at the United Nations summit on climate change, as well as many other international events with some of the world's most powerful leaders. She is an amazing example of the impact one person can have. In front of global governments filled with those old enough to be her parents, her grandparents, or even her great-grandparents, Greta stood up for something she believed in and is making a difference.

2

FEEL

AMAZING

YOU WILL PERSONALLY BENEFIT

One of the best things about being vegan is that, in some poetic twist of fate, the very thing that can save our planet is also a better way to live. The chances are you will feel better on a plant-based diet. It can help you live a longer, happier, healthier life, while still delivering all the deliciousness that you're used to. It can be cheaper and easier, too.

This might just be the best decision that you ever made.

We met an Uber driver once after a supper club we hosted. He was one of the most smiley men you'll ever meet. But he told us a story. Five years ago, his sinusitis was so bad it was making his life impossible. He had tried everything. He couldn't breathe. He couldn't sleep. His face was on fire and his eyes were constantly streaming. Nothing worked and quite simply he didn"t know what to do. He was miserable and at his wits" end. Someone suggested he try a vegan diet, but he ignored the idea. His suffering was so bad that it was seriously affecting his life, as well as his friends and family. Life couldn't go on like this. He even considered ending it. Then he decided he might as well *try* going vegan.

He cut out meat, dairy, fish, and eggs and switched to a diet based on whole foods and colorful vegetables. Within weeks his sinusitis cleared up. He felt better than he had in years. Over the following years he lost weight and shared his story and his transformation with everyone. Most important, he discovered a new way of living and eating. Stories such as this are really common.

We are constantly messaged by people who have seen incredible health benefits and recoveries from poor health following a switch to a plant-based diet. Whether it's recovery from asthma or obesity, we have been told dozens of stories like our Uber driver's. Ask around and you won't have any trouble finding loads of anecdotal evidence for how much better you feel when you switch to vegan eating.

We can also echo that view. We felt AMAZING almost as soon as we cut out meat and dairy. Within days, we both felt like we'd discovered a superpower, a new feeling of lightness, a new energy that we didn't have before. We still feel that way today; we've never looked back.

The 3 p.m. lull in energy? Not a thing anymore. That feeling after you've eaten too much fatty food? That's gone, too. Feeling slow and lethargic in the morning? That doesn't happen now. Henry's crippling hay fever pretty much disappeared as well. Before, he used to spend the summer months in misery—streaming eyes, sneezing, feeling tired all the time . . . popping antihistamines every day. Now, he has maybe four or five days a year when he might suffer due to a very high pollen count. Choosing vegan was the best decision of our lives.

So that's the good news. And we think it's pretty awesome news. The one thing that we can all do to reduce the damage to our planet, and maybe even reverse climate change, is also an incredibly powerful change to make for ourselves. One that may make you feel better than ever before.

You can have your cake and eat it. As long as it's vegan cake.

YOU'LL BE
HEALTHIER, TOO

It is ironic that some people criticize the vegan diet for being unhealthy, when the standard, Western way of eating is much less healthy! Highly processed, high in fats, low in fruit and veg . . . In today's world of high cholesterol levels and high blood pressure, a plant-based diet is the best way to lower cholesterol. Plants are completely free from cholesterol. [68]

On a vegan diet you're eating an incredibly diverse range of plant foods on a regular basis. It's one of the things that makes sticking to a vegan diet so easy—you get to explore and enjoy so many more amazing ingredients than you might if your diet was based around animal products. Plant-based cooking encourages us to be more adventurous and experimental with our food choices—and we love it!

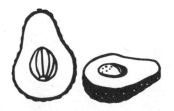

Plant-based foods, particularly fruit and vegetables, nuts, beans, and seeds, have been shown to help in the treatment of many chronic diseases and are often associated with lower rates of type 2 diabetes, less hypertension, lower cholesterol levels, and reduced cancer rates.[69]

DIABETES UK

Plant-based foods are rich in fiber, antioxidants, folate, and various phytochemicals, all of which are all great for our general health. Often a whole-foods, plant-based diet contains fewer calories, too, so it's easier to maintain a healthy body weight, and many people say that any excess weight just falls off (it did for us).

If you're worried about your energy levels or maintaining your performance at the gym, know that many world-class athletes have made the switch to a plant-based diet, including soccer players, basketball players, boxers, and tennis champs. They all claim better recovery from exercise and better digestion on a plant-based diet. But perhaps the most persuasive example of this is Patrik Baboumian, the German stongman competitor who has broken world records since becoming vegan. We applaud and admire these amazing, inspiring, ripped dudes and dudettes who are smashing it on a plant-based diet. We are so grateful to them!

There are countless studies to back up the fact that a balanced plant-based diet, or a mostly plant-based diet, is the best diet for your body—it can even reduce premature deaths from chronic diseases by more than 20%.[70] These are studies from objective bodies like the World Health Organization, United Nations,[71] Harvard University,[72, 73] Oxford University,[74] as well as progressive governments (for example, the Canadian government has removed dairy entirely from its list of recommended foods, which is now 90% plant-based).[75]

Processed meats and fish have now been linked to increased risk of **breast cancer**.[76] Eating red meat substantially raises your risk of death from cancer or heart disease.[77]

A plant-based diet is increasingly recognized as a healthier alternative. **Atherosclerosis**, or plaque in your arteries, associated with **high intake of meat, fat, and carbohydrates**, is the leading cause of death in the USA.[78]

The World Health Organization (WHO) has listed **red meat** and **processed meat** as **carcinogenic**.[79]

The US FDA advises that some **fish and shellfish** can contain unpredictable and potentially damaging levels of **mercury**, and are now deemed unadvisable for pregnant women, breastfeeding mothers, or children.[80]

By eating a plant-based diet you can save the planet, and be healthier, too.

The principles of
a healthy diet are
simple: eat whole,
colorful, mostly
plant-based foods,
including quality fats
and plenty of fiber.

DR. RUPY AUJLA
Eat to Beat Illness

FEEL CLEAN

A plant-based diet is also really clean! The main foods that are likely to be contaminated if not handled, stored, or cooked properly are raw meat and poultry, raw eggs, raw shellfish, unpasteurized milk, and ready-to-eat foods like deli meats, pâtés, and soft cheeses.[81] Not plants. To put it bluntly, if you get food poisoning from animal products, it's bad luck. If you get food poisoning from plant-based foods, then generally it's because someone in the kitchen has not washed their hands properly.[82]

By contrast, coliform bacteria, which are used as a marker for fecal contamination, typically find their way into your kitchen via meat, which is often contaminated with fecal bacteria.[83] Plant-based foods are inherently cleaner, and a plant-based kitchen is a cleaner kitchen.

The other thing that will be cleaner is your conscience. By choosing more plant-based foods you will know that you are living in a more sustainable way. This peace and clarity of mind is invaluable—something we both experienced when going vegan. The way we were eating synced with our values. We suddenly felt like everything made a bit more sense, and it helped inform a lot of the other decisions we made in our lives.

There is a new kind of consumer appearing, one who is more conscious of their health and the environment, one perfectly happy to make dietary changes, such as becoming vegan, vegetarian, or flexitarian to achieve those aims. Perhaps our friend Zanna Van Dijk, a fitness influencer who made the move to a plant-based diet, said it better than we can:

"Eating plant-based completely transformed my mindset, as finally my actions were in line with my values. I found myself more compassionate toward animals and humans and connecting more deeply with those around me.

"I found a new appreciation for the environment and a heightened sense of consciousness in all my actions and the impact they have on people and the natural world. I realized that I'm part of a bigger picture, my choices go far beyond myself, and that power comes with responsibility to be a good human."

IT'LL SAVE MONEY, TOO

Compared to a typical meat eater, vegetarians can save much more on food each year,[84] especially if you are comparing plant-based items with high-quality, organic, free-range meat. If you're looking to keep costs down, then we suggest avoiding processed, packaged "vegan" foods, and instead look to fill your plate with vegetables, grains, and home-cooked foods—which is, of course, the best way to eat for your health, too.

When we've been short of cash, we've both relied on forward planning. And we try to do that now, too, because it makes good sense (see page 230 for advice on how to meal plan). Ian remembers when he first moved to London. He was on a very low salary, thankful to be living and working in London, but after rent and bills were paid, he was left with very little money. He tracked his outgo and worked out pretty quickly that he was spending too much on food. Ian started to approach lunch like a fun challenge and gamified the process of designing budget lunches. The budget he set himself was five quid for five days. One pound a day. That might seem ridiculous but, as he says himself, "I'm from Yorkshire and frugality runs through my veins." With a little creativity, confidence, and the right attitude, eating on a budget is not only possible but actually, very satisfying. And it's just as easy as a vegan!

When we first went vegan we ate tons of pasta because it's cheap and filling. We practiced making loads of different pasta sauces, one of which, Easy Peasy Pasta, ended up in our first book and has now been made by folks all over the world!

Also . . . thinking long-term, with all that healthy fiber and masses of colored foods packed with health-giving nutrients, you're likely to save money on healthcare and medication in later life, too. Your body will be in much better shape. In fact, in the UK, billions could be saved from the country's annual health bill if more people followed a plant-based diet. [85]

ARM YOUR BULLSHIT DETECTOR...

. . . and be prepared to take it everywhere you go.

A plant-based diet, and the vegan movement in general, has had so much negative press that, when you start telling people you're vegan, you will encounter judgment disguised as advice. Some of it may even seem like useful information.

We've all heard stories of people who avoid doctors. And we've all seen influencers on social media promoting the latest diet, health, or fitness trend with no supervision. Never take health and nutrition advice from unqualified people! And don't be afraid of doctors. Doctors are great. They are there to help you.

Now, of course, doctors don't always get things right. In fact, historically there has not been enough nutritional training given during their studies, although people like our friends Dr. Rupy Aujla of *The Doctor's Kitchen* or Hazel Wallace of *The Food Medic* are working to change that! But in the past, and still in many GP practices, doctors may be overly cautious when it comes to vegan diets. However, doctors are trained in the art of medicine. Real medicine. They have an excellent understanding of your body and your health and they literally swear an oath to help you.

So use them! If you have any questions about your health or your diet, then seek medical advice. You might even be able to find a plant-based or vegan doctor who can give you even more targeted advice. Look after yourself. If you're still in doubt, seek a second opinion. But a second *medical* opinion (not a friend's).

You may also seek advice from other professionals, such as dieticians or nutritionists. However, be aware that all are not created equally and always check the credentials of the people you choose. It's possible to get a nutritionist's certificate from the internet with little to no experience. Look for accredited, credible professionals with clear evidence of clients, real testimonials, and papers published. Speak to them before you engage them, suss them out, and ask to speak to reference clients.

Advice is just that, advice.
Ask questions, listen to your gut,
and keep learning.

Vegan may not be the only way, but it's a good way.
There is no one optimum human diet. On the island of
Okinawa in Japan, people eat a predominantly plant-based
diet, but with a small amount of fish and other meats.[86]
The Okinawan diet is largely viewed as one of the
healthiest ways to eat.

A balanced vegan diet is not the only diet that will give you
the best chances of living the longest. But it's certainly up
there with the best. And it's easy.

It's easy because there's a simple set of rules, which we'll
come to in the next part of the book. And by following them
you will know that you are giving your body the best chance.
It's easier than calorie counting, meal tracking, macro
crunching, or meat restricting. Just one simple "no"—the "no"
to consuming animal products—is all that's required.

Science tells us that a vegan diet can help us prevent or
even reverse diseases, living longer, happier, healthier lives.
And, most important, it's also the best way we know to tackle
climate change. Putting plants on your plate means you
are doing the best thing to protect your body and save the
planet.

All of this
comes from just
one simple choice.
Say "no" to animals
on your plate to
feel better in your
body and save
our planet.

(3)

YOU
CAN
DO IT

BUMPS IN THE ROAD TO WATCH OUT FOR

BALANCE

A well-planned plant-based diet is thought to be one of the best diets for human and planetary health. But just like any diet, it can also be unhealthy. French fries and Oreos are vegan, too! Our key advice when following a plant-based or vegan diet is to eat the rainbow. Eat plenty of colorful plant whole foods, and avoid beige, processed carbohydrates. With a bit of forward planning, a vegan diet can be beneficial for people at all stages of life.

Contrary to what you may have heard, many nutritional deficiencies are much less common in people who eat a varied plant-based diet rather than a standard Western diet.[87] A diet built on a variety of beans, greens, whole grains, fruits, and vegetables is naturally packed with all the fiber, potassium, magnesium, vitamins, antioxidants, and protein that your body needs to thrive! Not to mention this nice little bonus: plants contain zero cholesterol. If you don't believe us, maybe you'll believe the American Academy of Nutrition and Dietetics (the world's biggest professional body for registered dieticians and nutrition professionals). In their considered opinion, vegetarian and vegan diets are "healthful, nutritionally adequate, and may provide health benefits in the prevention and treatment of certain diseases."[88] Plant-based diets have also been endorsed by the British Dietetic Association as healthy for people of all ages.[89] But please remember that we're not nutritionists or doctors. If you have concerns about your health, consult a healthcare professional.

It is possible to get all the nutrients you need on a vegan diet from eating a good variety of plants, with one exception: vitamin B12. This is because B12 is made by soil bacteria, and these days our food and water are (thankfully) usually clean and soil-free. As animals do consume some soil, or are given supplements, meat does contain vitamin B12. This isn't just a vegan issue—a whopping 39% of people are low in vitamin B12.[90] However, it's now really easy to get enough B12 by consuming fortified milks, nutritional yeast, or a regular supplement.

However, there are some nutrients that are more readily available in animal products, so you will need to ensure you are eating adequate amounts of these, including calcium and omega-3 fatty acids. It's also important to get enough iron, zinc, and vitamin D.[91] Everyone can be deficient in these, not just vegans.

People often worry about calcium. Make sure you drink plenty of fortified plant-based milk and eat green leafy veg. Likewise iron, which can be found in whole grains, nuts and seeds, beans, and green veg, so pack your diet with these!

As backup, so we don't constantly track everything we eat, we take a daily multivitamin—you can even get ones designed with vegans in mind now. We also eat flaxseeds and chia seeds for their omega-3s, and we occasionally take an algae-based omega-3 supplement. We may also use a vitamin D spray if we feel we haven't seen the sun for a while . . .

All diets come with their own things to consider: the typical Western diet is notoriously low in dietary fiber [92] and many people need to be aware of the risk of higher cholesterol, while the Mediterranean diet can come with a risk of increased mercury due to its high intake of fish. [93] Cheesy pizza is a really good source of calcium, but we all know that a diet based around pizza isn't going to be good for you, even if you're hitting those calcium goals. Like everything, you just have to be sensible.

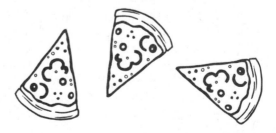

OTHER PEOPLE . . .

Your family and friends may not agree with your choices and this can be difficult to navigate at times. It definitely makes vegan eating much easier, especially in the early stages, if you are able to try it out as a group, so it's worth seeing if anyone wants to join you. Maybe you can all try Veganuary together, or even have a vegan week or do meat-free Mondays. If they want to give it a go, then great. But if not, that's OK, too. It's good to speak up for what you believe in, but it's a fact of life that everyone is on their own journey, and we can't all think the same as each other.

Sadly, it's not uncommon for friends and family to challenge your decision to go vegan—or even just your plan to adopt a more plant-based diet. We've experienced the whole spectrum of reactions, from interested and supportive comments, to expressions of disgust and full-blown arguments. We had one waitress, in London, stick her tongue out and blow a disapproving raspberry noise at us when we told her we were vegan! It means different things to different people, and by moving toward vegan eating you'll be finding yourself in uncharted territory.

IAN'S STORY

When I first went vegan, I told my family and they were like, "OK, cool, you do you." They were reasonably blasé about the idea. After a month they asked, "Have you stopped with that vegan thing yet?" I replied, "Erm, no, I'm still very much 'doing that vegan thing' and, to be honest, I think I'll be doing it for a fair while yet." After another month, my family seemed to be reasonably concerned about health and general well-being. My mum, who's a nurse, would say things like, "You need to stop this now, it's not healthy, you need meat for protein and you need milk for calcium." To her credit, she had my best interests at heart, and she was genuinely concerned about me. After all, "this vegan thing" was completely and totally out of sync with the way I had been brought up.

I remember having a conversation with my mum about my decision to go vegan. She told me it felt like a kick in the teeth for her because veganism is completely different from the way I was raised. I completely sympathize with how she must have felt and appreciate that initially it must have been quite a difficult thing to grasp. Now, even though my parents aren't vegan, they're a lot more conscious of what they're eating. They're much more open to the idea of vegetarian food and are very happy to text and tell me when they've eaten a vegan or veggie meal! And I love to hear about it. Time was definitely the most important factor in my parents accepting I'm in "this vegan thing" for the long haul.

Friends and family are really important, so our main piece of advice is, if possible, to keep your family and friends as family and friends. Try not to end up in huge arguments, disown them, or cause them to disown you. Everyone's on their own path. What's true for you is not necessarily true for them, so don't make the mistake of judging everyone by your own standards, and you will find it easier to exist in a world with differing views and opinions. Live and let live—you might be surprised how many people start to join you.

Be a happy, friendly, positive advertisement for veganism. If you're vegan, or vegan-ish, don't be afraid to hang out with people who aren't. Just be a shining beacon of inspiration to all you meet.

DATING A NONVEGAN

Dating people with different dietary preferences can be challenging, but it doesn't need to be. Since we went vegan, we've both dated people who have been meat eaters. Obviously being in the vegan scene and frequenting vegan events, we end up socializing with a lot of vegan people. Going on dates with people who are also vegan is great, because you automatically have a big part of your life in common and shared beliefs.

Henry is now engaged to EmJ, who is vegan. They met in a corridor while Henry was helping buddies JP and Alex with their new food company. Henry says, "I walked through the corridor, looking all cool, carrying my motorcycle helmet, and helped her carry her bags up the stairs. Schmooove. She was already vegan, which was a real conversation starter. Life's so much easier because we're both vegan. We can make joint decisions whether eating at home, out, or on holiday."

Ian says, "Dating nonvegans is fab because conversation is always boundless. I've been on dates where I've answered questions about why I'm vegan the entire evening. Some people aren't that keen on the idea of dating a vegan—but some love it! In fact, one of the women I dated, who I now consider a friend, messaged me to say: 'Today is my one-year veganniversary . . . So thank you. Best life choice ever!'"

OUR TIPS FOR DEALING WITH OTHER PEOPLE

When eating with family and friends, make an extra effort to help things run really smoothly. If you're going to a restaurant, phone ahead or check the menu online. If you're going to someone's home for dinner, chat with the host in advance to check what you can eat. Perhaps offer to bring a dish yourself, or if they are willing, suggest a recipe that they can cook. It's worth doing as much of this as possible before the event, so you can avoid any awkward moments. Your goal is to make it look easy and make everyone feel comfortable. This will give the most powerful impression of how easy and simple it is to live a normal life and eat vegan food. (See pages 232–239 for more on eating out.)

Another thing to get ready to accept is a little bit of gentle teasing.

Depending on your friendship group, you may have some people who make fun of you. We certainly do. It's fine. It happens and it's a part of life. Sometimes people will make fun of what they don't understand, and they probably don't realize it can be offensive. Try to let gentle jokes wash over you, as you know what you are doing is for you, not for them. It's best not to overreact or react at all. However, while a little bit of light-hearted banter is one thing, if you find you are being bullied, then it may be time to find some new friends!

If you live with nonvegans, always be respectful. Remember that even if you believe in something wholeheartedly, it doesn't mean that other people do.

Don't preach

When you discover new information and feel passionate about a cause, it can be so tempting to share what you have learned with those around you. This might be called "preaching," "judging," or "lecturing," and it's a really easy trap to fall into as a new vegan.

We have certainly been guilty of this. When we first became vegan, we were so shocked by what was going on in the world that we had to tell all our friends about it. We shared our reasons with everyone, and in a fairly forceful way. Unsurprisingly, we got mixed reactions!

"You've seen *Cowspiracy*, I've sent you links to a bunch of websites, we chatted about this at the pub last time I saw you and yet you're still eating animals. It's like you just don't care!" This is the kind of arrogant thing we probably said to our friends at one point or another. This patronizing and combative tone is really unhelpful and is likely to put people off veganism. (Huge apologies to anyone we talked to like this in the early days!)

Some were supportive, some were offended and argumentative. Some felt patronized. Some decided it would be funny to mock our dietary choices at every chance they got (remember Naushard?!). These are all different reactions that you might encounter.

That's why we set up **BOSH!**, and it's why the channel has been successful. We're not preachy or judgmental, and we make food for everybody—vegans, veggies, and flexis alike. We answer people's questions when asked, but we do so in a way that we hope is informed but also informal, relatable, and relaxed.

If people ask you a question, give an answer that avoids being judgmental. Focus on your own choices, rather than pushing your views onto them.

TRICKY QUESTIONS PEOPLE MIGHT ASK YOU

1 **You say you're vegan because you care about the environment. Why do you think it's OK to fly to America?**

It's as important to fill life with experience, excitement, and adventure as it is to live it with kindness, concern, and love. The conversations you have with people on your adventures might inspire them to think differently about the way they live their life, perhaps motivating them to make positive choices that will affect the world in a beneficial way.

2 **I've seen a picture of you on Facebook wearing a leather jacket. I thought you were supposed to be vegan?**

You can't change the past but you can affect the future. I'll think carefully about leather from now on, but we shouldn't be wasteful with the clothes we have.

3 **This taxi has leather seats. I thought you were vegan?**

I'll control my environment to the best of my ability. If I ever buy a car, I'll make sure it doesn't have leather seats, but right now this taxi is going to get me home safe and sound.

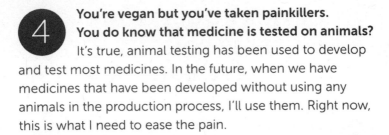

4 **You're vegan but you've taken painkillers. You do know that medicine is tested on animals?** It's true, animal testing has been used to develop and test most medicines. In the future, when we have medicines that have been developed without using any animals in the production process, I'll use them. Right now, this is what I need to ease the pain.

5 **You don't eat meat but you have an iPhone. What about the conditions of the people that mine the minerals and metal? Don't they matter?** The people who mined the materials to make this phone matter. Of course they do. I'm extremely grateful to them and appreciate their hard work. We need to look at every aspect of modern society and make some fundamental changes. We used the tools that were available to us (cameras and social media) to set up **BOSH!** and do our bit. Everyone who has a smartphone now has a pocketful of possibility and the opportunity to make change and do good.

Sometimes people may raise questions that you don't know the answer to or make points that you haven't thought about. It can occasionally seem way too complicated. In a world where our biggest threat is something as big and hard to understand as climate change, there are many possible right answers.

Don't get lost in debates or arguments; you know why you are vegan, and you don't need anyone's approval.

At the beginning of our vegan journey, we were easily annoyed and frustrated when people asked questions. However, we realized we were only getting so annoyed because we didn't know the answers. Because we were in this for the long haul, we needed to be able to answer questions with confidence. So we read articles and memorized numerous facts. Now, we love talking to people about veganism; it's a great opportunity to articulate our own thoughts, process ideas, and ultimately talk about our favorite subject.

More on this and some answers to common questions, on pages 302–307.

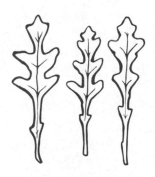

FINDING YOUR TRIBE

In this day and age, with millions of people moving toward more environmentally friendly, healthy, plant-based diets, you no longer risk being made fun of for your food choices! Make some new friends by joining local events, volunteering, or just finding new social circles.

When we first went vegan, we didn't know many people who were doing it, too. So we threw ourselves into the vegan scene in London.

We went to every event, and got really involved in Vevolution—an amazing global organization that champions all aspects of plant-based eating and living. We went to master classes on sustainable fashion and activism, and we hung out with people after the events; we met the guys behind Veganuary and Allplants, and fully immersed ourselves in this new group.

It's so important to find some like-minded people who you can share this journey with. There are plenty of online communities of course, but if you make the effort in real life you will feel so much more connected and supported. See what's going on near you and join in the fun!

HAVE STRONG OPINIONS THAT ARE WEAKLY HELD

A venture capitalist from California, Marc Andreessen, introduced us to the phrase "strong opinions, weakly held." Much wisdom lies in these four words.

Have you ever met someone opinionated, who is prone to change at the drop of a hat? Would you take that person's advice on anything? Having weak opinions is a terrible way to go about life, and could be exhausting, as you're constantly questioning yourself. Conversely, though, have you ever met someone who is so opinionated that they dig their heels in, despite overwhelming evidence, stubbornly sticking to their version even if you suspect they no longer believe it themselves?

HENRY, ON FINDING HIS TRIBE

When I moved to London at age 22, I remember it being a very lonely experience. I lived with friends but knew very few other people. I worked in digital and marketing and had work friends, but still found London to be a lonely place. As a start-up founder, I had a team full of people—30 at its biggest—but despite being surrounded by people, and even having a few friends (including Ian) in the team, there was an incredible amount of pressure on my shoulders and I found it really isolating. After a moment of clarity I made the decision to pursue a life that involved building a business with meaning and purpose and changing the way I looked at the world.

With that new perspective came new people, people with more integrity. Ian and I embarked on building a business that was completely focused on doing good in the world. We vowed to act with complete integrity in everything we did and to surround ourselves with people who had similar beliefs and passions.

We immersed ourselves into the London vegan community and the London food scene. We made good friends with those who ran vegan events, and went to networking and social events, even if we didn't feel like it.

Wherever we could we helped those in need. We built a team of like-minded people who are honest, trustworthy, and talented and who want to work with us on our mission to change the world for the better.

Over the last four years, I've been anything but lonely. I'm surrounded by people I trust, who believe in me and who I believe in, too. I live in a shared house with Ian, my fiancée, EmJ, and our friend Anna, who is also vegan and shares our morals and ideals. We've got great friends within the vegan community—from mentors and mentees to advisors. We've even been to a few vegan weddings. From a personal perspective we've also never been healthier.

Finding my tribe has been incredibly important, taking me from a largely solitary place to a social and well-connected one, surrounded by allies, all trying to change the world for the better.

Decide what your values are, make them a core part of your being, and then align yourself with people who share your perspective. We all need people around us to help us succeed in our lives, so find those people for you.

Make your decisions slowly and with consideration.
Do your research. Spend time thinking through your
reasons—it can be helpful to write them down. Plan how
you are going to do it. You've made a carefully considered
decision, based on all the available facts; don't let a
whimsical conversation or comment throw you off track.
Don't let a family member question your entire stance on
climate change because you fly once a year. Don't let badly
researched newspaper articles convince you that vegans
are unhealthy.

Don't lose your flexibility.
Keep learning. Remain open
to new ideas. Stay humble.

Listen to advice. Take comments on board and do your own
research. Don't be that person who won't listen to anyone
around them. Be prepared to learn. Be flexible. But also learn
to weed out bad advice. And watch out for bad science—
there are plenty of people peddling claims that are based on
poor research.

DO IT YOUR WAY

As we've already said, as you start to make some decisions about how to live a vegan life, it's important to realize that there is no one-size-fits-all solution.

Even the word "vegan," which is seemingly about one set of choices, is actually subject to countless variations in meaning. Veganism is an ideal, but it is not about perfection. If you, right now, were to eat vegan 80% of the time, the impact on your personal carbon footprint would be huge. You would positively impact animal welfare and you would likely see a diet-dependent improvement in your health, too. All you can do is identify how you can apply the ideas of being vegan to your life.

That's not to say we thought like this from the outset. When we first went vegan, we were very excited about our new life choices and we wanted to share it with everyone! Unsurprisingly, sometimes people just didn't want to hear why we'd made this decision. We made lots of missteps and probably unintentionally upset people in the process. Our advice to you is to avoid debates. Know that sometimes there really isn't a right or wrong answer, so the best thing you can do is let it slide.

Today we're able to eat vegan food at nearly every single restaurant we go to, find vegan sausages and ice cream in many shops (Henry's favorite is chocolate and nut, and Ian's is vanilla, in case you're wondering). This is thanks to meat eaters. It sounds crazy, but it's true. Because people are choosing to eat more plant-based meals—not necessarily going fully vegan—the demand for vegan food is high. Wherever you are on your journey, eating more plant-based foods makes it easier for other people to be vegan.

Show other people how great it is to eat a more plant-based diet. Cook food for people. Share your food photos on your social media channels (if you use our recipes, then tag us!). Go to social events and talk about your choices in a positive, warm, nonjudgmental manner. Doing this, you can have an incredible impact on those around you, affecting their social circles, too—and so veganism will reach more and more people, encouraging them to switch to a more plant-based way of life.

And that's it.
It's actually
really simple.

NOW IT'S YOUR TURN

So, we've shared our journey with you. But everybody is different. The questions on these pages are a chance for you to reflect on why you're trying a vegan diet, and how you think you'll achieve it.

DEFINE YOUR WHY

At this stage, it can be useful to think about why you are choosing to make this change. Maybe even write it down. Setting it all down can bring clarity, and you can revisit your statements later to help keep you motivated if you ever need to remind yourself why you are doing this. Here are some questions to get you started:

Why did you pick up this book?

Why are you looking to make a change?

What's your motivation for eating a more plant-based diet?

What is your goal? What would you like to achieve?

What core belief is motivating you to change?

What change do you want to see in the world?

What will be easy?

What will be difficult?

What will you miss?

How will you feel when/if people question your decision?

What will you say to those people?

It's important to identify why you are choosing to adopt a more vegan lifestyle. Note down how you think these changes will make you feel, both good and bad, so you can be prepared for the ups and downs.

DEFINE YOUR HOW

As with everything, a little advance planning can make all the difference when trying to create a new habit or creating a lifestyle change. We went vegan overnight—and it's not at all difficult to do, especially these days—but making an action plan for how you are going to make plant-based eating fit into your life will help make the transition easier. Setting a few basic rules for yourself will help keep you on track.

Are you going to eat vegan meals every day? A few days a week? Every morning? Or just on weekdays? Meat-free Mondays, perhaps?

How strict are you going to be? Are you all in from day one, or trying a more phased approach?

Remind yourself of your goal in the previous section. How will you work toward this?

Is there anything that you are worried about not fitting into your new plant-based life? How will you tackle this?

Are you going to be fully vegan, for example buy vegan products, toiletries and clothes, or start with a vegan diet?

Who will help you stay motivated? Who are your allies? Your tribe?

How do you feel when you think about making this big change?

How will you feel when you have achieved your goal?

What are you worried about?

How will you overcome this?

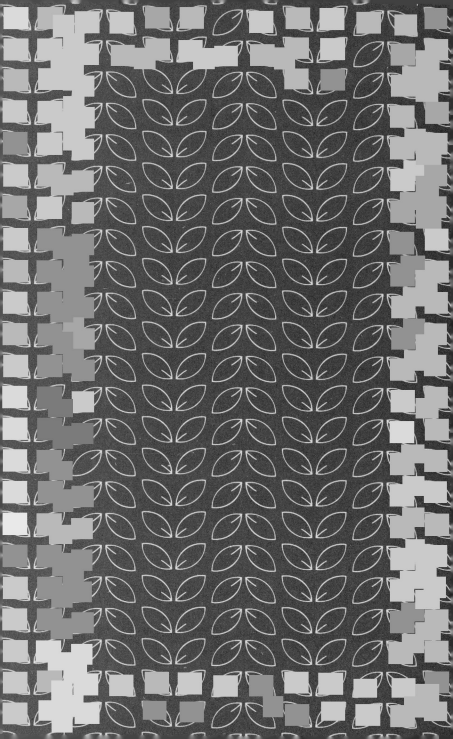

HOW?

Eat food, not too much, mostly plants.

MICHAEL POLLAN
Food Rules: An Eater's Manual

It's now easier than it's ever been to eat plant-based meals.

There's an unbelievable amount of choice these days, with supermarket chains and restaurants proudly shouting about their veggie and vegan options and seeing their sales skyrocket as a result! Even just a few years ago when we started our vegan journey, it would be difficult to find good options. In the first few months, we'd nip into a supermarket to grab some lunch and stand there picking up random sandwiches, checking all the labels. Every sandwich was vegan-unfriendly. We became desperate, picking up random sandwiches one by one, slowly realizing that none were for us.

Premade sandwiches are now infinitely better than they used to be! Today the main problem we have is "Which one shall I pick?!" As more people adopt a plant-based diet, the demand for quality vegan and veggie products has grown at an incredible rate, and this means the options are also increasing every day.

One-third of Brits,[94] meaning about **12 million people**, are now vegan, veggie, or flexitarian (flexitarians are those who follow a mainly plant-based diet, eating meat only occasionally). That's a huge number moving away from animal products and toward a veggie diet.

Even meat eaters are reducing the amount of meat they eat.[95] In the US, sales of plant-based alternatives to meat, cheese, milk, and eggs increased by **17%** in just one year,[96] and sales of meat-substitutes have **doubled** in the last five years.[97]

The vegan milk company Oatly has seen "hyper growth in demand," and a **60%** increase in turnover in one year, as more people move away from dairy in their hot drinks.[98] The creator of the faux-meat burger Beyond Meat soared **163%** in the biggest US IPO since the year 2000.[99] When UK sandwich shop Greggs launched their Vegan Sausage Roll in January 2019, its shares rose more than **10%**—a record high.[100] Investors and retailers are aware that vegan and vegetarian food is the biggest growth area, and the demand will continue to increase, if not accelerate, over the coming years.[101] [102]

So, while the media like to portray "mad militant vegans" and "angry farmers" arguing with each other, the reality is exactly the opposite: **everyone is getting a bit more plant-based.**

We're here to show you how to eat more plants—or fewer animals—and how to apply the same thinking to the rest of your life, too.

We want to show you how it's possible to eat vegan (or mostly vegan) food and still keep your friends and your social life! We've distilled what we've learned from our years building and maintaining social media channels with more than 2.5 million active, opinionated, vegan, veggie, flexi, and meat-eating subscribers.

Michael Pollan said it best, when he summarized his book *Food Rules: An Eater's Manual* into the phrase "eat food, not too much, mostly plants." We think this is a perfect mantra.

SO, WHAT CAN I EAT?

Before we decided to go plant-based, we both ate a really traditional Western-style diet. Every single meal was based around some kind of animal protein. We loved our eggs and bacon for breakfast, lunches usually consisted of cheese or ham sandwiches, and our dinner plates were typically a big piece of protein with some token veg.

No wonder we weren't getting enough fruits and veggies a day! We were getting our protein, sure, but there wasn't nearly enough color on our plates. Far too many of our "vegetable" portions consisted of potatoes, whether roasted, mashed, or deep-fried.

At first, we worried that cutting out animal products would be massively restrictive. What would we replace them with?!

Would we ever be able to eat our favorite foods again?

In particular, we were worried about losing fry-ups and big, hearty breakfasts! That's why we started creating our own dishes, mastering cooking—we wanted to re-create vegan versions of the dishes we missed the most. Basing your meals around lots of different types of veg actually means you can eat so much more imaginatively. We think our food is much more interesting and tastier now.

Our approach to food today follows the mantra "eat the rainbow," and we aim to include as much variety as we possibly can.

That's not to say we don't ever eat meals that look "traditional." We've made plant-based versions of fish and chips, lasagnas, roast dinners, curries, and more. And if we go to a festival or a street food market, we'll be eating burgers like in the old days—they'll just be plant-based ones now, with some melty, stringy vegan cheese on top . . .

We think our dishes are better **BOSH!**-style than the originals. We've been told that our cauliflower Buffalo wings are better than meaty ones, which have all the gross chicken-y bits and bones that you have to discard. Our wings are 100% edible!

And our spaghetti Bolognese—or really anything we make with minced mushroom—is at least as good as the original. With the added benefit of being cholesterol- and growth-hormone-free.

Our diet now includes such a broad range it's impossible to compare it to our old ways.

Even if some of the meals look the same, the overall picture is very different. We are just as satisfied with a well-put-together Buddha bowl as we were with the classic meat and two veg.

As you eat more plant-based foods, you may find that your plates look different. Some of your meals may be more like picnics or consist of sharing plates—like Spanish tapas or Middle Eastern mezze. You'll discover that celery, hummus, and various dippy bits (technical term!) can constitute a healthy, filling, and nutritious lunch.

When we first cut out meat and dairy, we went cold turkey (excuse the pun). We cut out everything. We read the labels of everything in our kitchen and removed all the foods that contained animal products. It took approximately half a day, but it made everything easier.

We also took some time to get to know our supermarket again, wandering around and looking at products, and asking a lot of people a lot of questions. We made false steps, for sure, and four years into our journey our knowledge is still not perfect. But our decision was firm, and we've learned a lot about food and nutrition.

Animal products can end up in many places you wouldn't expect. Snack foods in particular are an easy place to get caught out. In the early days we'd often find ourselves halfway through a bag of potato chips before finding out they contained some kind of powdered milk.

Now we know instinctively which sections of the supermarket to head to, which products to buy, and which to avoid—and how to **BOSH!** our favorite meaty meals, making them plant-based. We've developed that knowledge, and now we want to share it with you.

to **BOSH!** *verb*: to veganize a dish in the most delicious way

OUR 5 GOLDEN RULES

A plant-based diet is packed full of things that are incredibly good for you, and can be one of the healthiest diets you can follow. Yes, there are a few things to be conscious of: as with any way of eating, we need to ensure that we get the right nutrient balance in our bodies. Thinking about nutrition is a good thing though, and something that everyone should do, whether they're vegan, veggie, flexi, or mindfully meaty.

1

EAT THE RAINBOW

When we put together a plate of food, we roughly aim for it to be made up of 50% fruits and veggies, 25% whole grains, and 25% plant-based protein: the 50/25/25 rule. This is also broadly in line with the NHS Eatwell Plate, Canadian Food Plate, and Vegan Power Plate. We call it the rainbow ratio, and it's an easy way to aim for a balanced diet—no laborious weighing or measuring of ingredients or portion sizes. It will ensure you are getting loads of fruits and veggies in your life on a daily basis, and adequate amounts of protein and grains without any fuss.

2

—

MIX UP YOUR PLATE

At every meal, as well as varying the colors, think about different textures, spices, and seasonal foodstuffs to give your body a broad range of vitamins and minerals. Mixing different protein sources across the day will also mean you'll get all the protein you need (see page 140 for more on plant-based protein).

3

—

EAT YOUR GREENS

Your parents always told you to eat your greens and they weren't wrong!

Get as much dark green in as you can, turbo-charging your daily diet with kale- and spinach-rich green smoothies. Anything dark green is packed with micronutrients that your body loves, so gorge on them. We like to kick-start every day with a massive green smoothie—see our recipe on page 188. It's such a great way to get ahead on your plant-based goodness!

4

—

THE 80/20 BALANCE

Follow the 80/20 rule: 80% healthy and 20% whatever you fancy. It's OK to eat a more unhealthy option from time to time, especially if it's home-cooked. Just balance it out with healthful and colorful foods the rest of the time. Food is there to be enjoyed! It plays a huge part in our culture, in our family lives, and in our sense of well-being, so it's really important to find a way of eating that fits within your life and makes you feel good. Maybe you will decide to eat healthily in the week and ease off on the weekend? Whatever works for you. See pages 230–231 for more on meal planning for the week and our best tips and tricks.

5

—

GET YOUR VITAMINS IN

We like to back up all our good eating with a daily multivitamin and B12 booster. That takes away any worry about hitting our nutrition goals. Take responsibility for learning some basic nutrition and, if you have concerns, think about checking with your doctor to make sure all's as it should be.

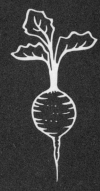

INGREDIENTS

"NO" FOODS

BASICALLY ALL ANIMAL PRODUCTS

OK, this is pretty obvious, which is why this list is fairly short compared with the lists on the following pages. Yes, a lot of the food served in restaurants and on the supermarket shelves are based around meat, fish, eggs, or cheese, so it can seem like there are a lot of things we're missing out on. But the actual number of foodstuffs that we avoid is relatively small, compared to the incredibly vibrant plethora of plant foods available! Whether you're going totally meat-free or sometimes-meat-free, these are the foods you'll be skipping.

Just think: "No animals, bits of animals or animal by-products."

Don't worry if you see some of your favorite food items here (we know how much people struggle with giving up cheese!)— we'll cover all the amazing alternatives now available on the following pages. You won't be missing out, we promise.

Meat and poultry, e.g., lamb, pork, beef, ground meat, chicken, duck, goose, turkey—anything that has a heart or central nervous system. This also includes processed versions of the above, such as ham, bacon, chorizo, etc.

Fish and seafood, e.g., all types of fish, tuna, shrimp, scallops, squid, mussels, crab, lobster, or anything that contains fish sauce (a liquid seasoning used in a lot of Asian cooking that is made from fermented fish).

Dairy products Anything that comes from the milk of a cow, goat, sheep, or any other animal, e.g., milk, cheese, yogurt, butter, ice cream, cream, buttermilk, whey, etc.

Eggs Whether they are from chickens, ducks, geese, fish, quails, or any other source. And this includes anything that contains eggs, e.g., mayonnaise, cakes, meringues, Hollandaise sauce, egg pasta, etc.

Honey or any other bee-derived products
This includes bee pollen and beeswax. Although farming bees doesn't necessarily kill them, it has a huge effect on the health of the bee and the hive—so it isn't vegan.

Any food products that contain any of the above ingredients, or derivatives of them
So check the label of foods you're not sure about. This is easy, and just becomes a habit. See page 163 for more about checking labels.

If it is
not an
ingredient,
then
check the
ingredients.

"YES" FOODS

ALL PLANTS

These are our "yes" foods. All plants. No animals here. This list contains food that, in the right quantities, can constitute a perfectly balanced plant-based diet. Read through these pages and imagine how colorful a plant-based diet can be.

There's often the misconception that it's hard to live on a plant-based diet. That's simply not true. Eating plants is anything but restrictive.

There are so many foods, so many flavors, so many textures and combinations. Eating more plants can also be much more affordable because so much of what we eat comprises whole foods and fresh ingredients.

Here are our "yes" foods, all our **BOSH!** foods, all just plants.

FRUITS

Fruits are plants. Duh. There is a wonderful variety of fruits to choose from, and the health benefits are many. You can opt for fresh, dried, or frozen; the choice is almost limitless. From **apples** and **cherries** to **jackfruit** (which makes a great meaty substitute in some of our favorite dishes like pulled pork) and **pomegranate seeds** for sprinkling over salads, fruits are a brilliant way to add extra flavor and nutrients.

Mangoes are particularly popular in the **BOSH!** house— Henry makes a mean noodle salad with mango, cashews, bean sprouts, and a soy sauce/sesame oil dressing. **Avocados** (technically a fruit but I think we all agree we treat them more like veg!) are also one of our quick go-tos— mashed on toast, in salads, in creamy dressings . . . it's one of the most versatile vegan ingredients. But don't forget the humble **banana** either—in a milkshake, in ice cream, or as a quick snack, baked with some dark chocolate in the middle . . .

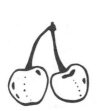 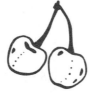

HENRY SAYS LEAVE AVOCADOS OUT OF IT!

Are avocados vegan? Well, some commentators have been quick to suggest not.

The reason, they explain, is because of the farming process called migratory beekeeping. Bees are taken around on trucks to pollenate plants, a process that could shorten the bees' lives and therefore cause suffering.

The Vegan Society was quick to confirm that avocados are considered vegan and to explain why: in today's society, it's difficult to eat foods that have not potentially caused harm to animals in some way. Modern farming practices will all have some effect on the animals that live in the surrounding area.[103]

This is a classic example of how some people are very quick to try to create an us vs. them positioning. People love to point out ways in which eating a vegan diet is unachievable, strengthening a dividing line and creating unnecessary "sides." This attitude is what we, at **BOSH!**, are devoted to removing.

We want everyone to enjoy eating more plants and appreciate plant-based food—we didn't even include the word "vegan" in our first cookbooks. And we want being vegan to be something that people can choose to do from time to time if they like. We all have to start somewhere!

VEGETABLES

Veggies are the core of what we eat. Fruit and veg make up about 50% of the perfect plant-based plate. There are so many amazing veg to choose from—from green **leafy veg**, to bright, sunshine yellow **peppers** and **squashes** to hearty winter **roots**.

Next time you go shopping, buy a vegetable you've not come across before and try it in your cooking.

The classic **eggplant** is one of our favorites—it's so versatile and has a great texture. There's nothing better than a big serving of salty roasted miso eggplant. We also love it in baba ganoush—an amazing smoky eggplant dip, which should be on every supermarket shelf next to hummus. We also make a lot of eggplant pickle—brinjal pickle—which goes wonderfully with a curry (or in a vegan cheese toastie).

LEGUMES

These include beans like **black beans** and **kidney beans**, which are perfect for dishes like chilis and stews. **Chickpeas** are one of our favorite legumes—they are the basis of the vegan staple hummus, and we also make falafel with them and add them to salads and curries. **Lentils** and **split peas** are incredibly versatile—and also cheap! Great for quick daals and soups.

HERBS AND SPICES

Ah, the delights of flavor! We love having a well-stocked dried spice drawer and herb rack. **Cilantro**, **parsley**, **rosemary**, and **basil** will always be on hand to bring dishes to life. The right combination of spices can work wonders, turning simple jackfruit, tofu, seitan, or tempeh into roasted dishes to rival the finest cuts of steak or chicken (see page 140 for more on our main meat replacements). And there's nothing like a fresh vegan pesto whizzed up in seconds to complement a simple bowl of spaghetti. Use fresh herbs wherever possible in curries, soups, or pasta dishes, and play around with spices, tasting and adjusting to get the perfect balance.

WHOLE GRAINS, FLOURS, PASTAS, RICE, COUSCOUS, AND NOODLES

Grains (and products derived from grains) form about a quarter of the perfect plant-based plate. **Oats** are a regular staple, as well as **rice**, and we're particular fans of **buckwheat noodles** and **pasta**. We always have a good loaf of bread in the house—made from wheat- or gluten-free flours, such as **rye**, **buckwheat**, or **corn**. **Chickpea flour** is super high in protein, tasty, and can be used for anything from chapatis to Indian pakoras to plant-based omelets. **Quinoa**, although technically a seed and not a grain, is a handy pantry ingredient to have as it is also a really good source of plant-based protein.

BAKING INGREDIENTS

We love baking! Luckily most baking ingredients are plant-based. We like to add extra flavor to our cakes and pastries with **vanilla extract**, **dried fruits**, **jams**, and **nuts**. If you're baking with **cocoa powder** or **chocolate**, check the label to make sure they're vegan. But do beware of **honey**—use maple syrup or agave nectar instead (see page 148).

HENRY'S CHOCOLATE CAKE

When my sister, Alice, and I were young, our parents totally spoiled us. They let us basically do whatever we wanted! Their freedom and belief in us set us up for life.

Every birthday, they would always cook this incredible cake. It was a family recipe, from my dad's side, handwritten in an old black notebook, packed in with a load of other recipes. A true family tradition.

The cake was wonderful: rich, indulgent, and super dark. In fact, dark chocolate gave it that kind of richness you only get with a good-quality chocolate bar, combined with incredible sweetness.

The cake was fluffy, perfectly moist, and topped with a huge layer of ganache-like chocolate icing. We called it the Devil's Cake and I can still remember the taste today.

When we went vegan, we struggled to find a vegan chocolate cake that could compare to this. So we needed to create one!

The same was true of my savory favorites, too, like lasagna and fish and chips. This search for irresistible vegan versions of all our old favorites was one of the reasons we set up **BOSH!**.

So we got to work in the kitchen. We made sure this cake had all the texture and sweetness I loved so much—even if the ingredients were different. And it was a hit!

At the time of writing this our Ultimate Chocolate Cake has had over 4 million views online. We get people coming up to us at every event telling us it's their favorite recipe. So we've literally shared my parents' secret recipe with the world! Sorry, folks, but it was worth it. The Devil's Cake was too Devilish to remain a secret!

SUGAR WARNING!

Typically, in the UK, sugar is vegan but in the US it often isn't, because animal bone char may have been used in the refining process. Whether or not to consider this vegan is a point of hot debate. If it's something you want to be sure about, then research vegan sugars in your local store or online.

You could also replace the sugar in your recipe with maple syrup. Replace every 230 g (1 cup) superfine sugar with 175 ml (¾ cup) maple syrup and reduce the other liquid content in the recipe by 3 tablespoons for every 240 ml (1 cup) maple syrup used.

In our opinion, if you want to hunt out vegan sugar, then go for it, but don't let decisions about the source of the sugar steer you away from eating an otherwise plant-based option.

NUTS AND SEEDS

We try to eat a good mix of nuts and seeds every day. They contain lots of different nutrients that are beneficial to the body, as well as healthy fats and proteins. The perfect vegan snack! Try filling a big jar with your favorite nuts and seeds and shake them about so they are well mixed.

Add a tablespoon of this to your morning granola, whip it up in your smoothies, or scatter it over salads. Do be aware that they are calorific—so a handful goes a long way! **Pumpkin seeds**, **flaxseeds**, and **chia seeds** are particularly nutritious.

In our minds, there's no better instant snack than PB&J on toast.

It's incredibly easy to make your own delicious nut butters—you can play around with adding spices, natural sweeteners, and even cocoa powder, too. And since we're talking about nuts, **cashews** are crucial in our cooking. We use blended cashews to make cream and milk replacements, in our béchamel, and for making cashew cheeses. Remember to soak them before blending to ensure they blitz down to a smooth cream, adding just a touch of water.

OILS AND VINEGARS

Oils and vinegars provide fats and acids for all our cooking, and are naturally vegan. We use **blended olive oils** for cooking, **extra-virgin olive oil** for finishing salads, and **sesame oil** for stir-fries. **Apple cider vinegar** is a regular in our cooking, and nothing beats **balsamic** on a salad or fresh bread. Do be aware though that oils are processed and very calorific, so don't overdo it.

MEAT AND DAIRY ALTERNATIVES

There are so many meat and dairy alternatives to choose from now—there has never been a better time to eat plant-based food! Whether it's the Beyond Burger or the Impossible Burger, Linda McCartney's sausages, or Good Catch tuna, there are ready-made alternatives to almost every meat. To find the best plant-based options, be prepared to experiment a little. Head to a big supermarket and test out a few. Check out your local natural foods store or get used to buying things online. With a small amount of effort, you'll see you can easily enjoy many of the things you used to love.

Here's a quick rundown of the most popular meat-alternative proteins:

Seitan
This is made from wheat gluten and is high in protein. It has a versatile texture and takes on flavor well. We recommend playing around with it to make vegan alternatives to things like hot wings, popcorn chicken, and chicken burgers.

Tempeh
This is the healthier cousin of seitan. It is less processed and, like tofu, it is made from soybeans. Tempeh has more texture than tofu, with some whole beans in the mix.

Tofu

This is the ingredient everyone thinks of when they imagine vegan cooking—and with good reason! We think tofu is amazing. It has a smooth texture as it's more finely processed than tempeh, and you can make so many delicious dishes with it. Our bacon-tofu slices recipe is still one of the most popular videos on our YouTube channel, and we make a mean salmon en croûte with tofu, too.

The only downside to these meat-replacement ingredients is that they are all processed. So see these as treats or occasional meals rather than everyday dinners, according to our 80/20 rule (see page 124).

A note on dairy-free dairy

There are some really impressive dairy-free milks and cheeses available now, too—and we like to make our own. Vegan cheeses can be quite variable, so try a few until you find a brand you like. We like the cheeses made by a company run by a friend of ours, called Kinda Co., or the Bute Island brand of cheeses in the UK. It's funny that we can put a man on the moon, but we can't yet make a perfect cheese without using a cow. But they're working on it!.

Nutritional yeast

We like to call this magic dust! These dried yeast flakes have a strong flavor, not unlike Parmesan. You can sprinkle it over finished dishes, use it to make a vegan cheese (see page 207), or add a little to stews and sauces to thicken.

Your plate has the power to change the planet.

LEARN TO BOSH! ANY RECIPE

Chances are, your favorite meals—the ones you cook most often—are probably meaty or cheesy. At some point you'll want to make them plant-based.

Maybe it's that perfect steak casserole, or that incredible cake. We're going to show you how to **BOSH!** it. That means removing the meat or dairy but saving the flavor, using a bit of culinary flair and some clever ingredient swaps.

We'll show you how you can make any recipe plant-based. Your friends and family might not even notice that it's vegan!

We count ourselves so lucky that our job is to "veganize" dishes. That's why we write our books: we want to make as many of our favorite meals available to everybody who wants to eat plant-based, whether for one day or every day.

Humans have been eating meat and animal products for thousands of years, so we've had incredible amounts of time to develop techniques based around milk, cheese, eggs, meats, and fish.

When you avoid these ingredients in your diet it forces you to innovate, to think of new ways to cook things, many of which have never been done before.

There's so much good stuff to discover, so much that's never been tasted before. That's what excites us.

Our creative process typically starts with choosing a favorite food or recipe, but one that isn't vegan, and we'll think about how to **BOSH!**ify it without using any animal products. But that's not enough—**BOSH!** isn't just about making meals vegan. The food needs to be fun, exciting, and accessible. So we'll design dishes that use ingredients that are easy to find. Then we'll taste-test the recipe and refine it again and again in the **BOSH!** kitchen until the flavor is where we want it. We'll refine and refine until it's perfect. Then it's time to make the video or put it in a book!

PRACTICE MAKES PERFECT

A word of warning: if you're **BOSH!**ing recipes, then you're in the world of experimentation, and just as you might invent something incredible . . . things can also go wrong! If you're in a high-pressure cooking situation (like when you've got six hungry folk waiting in the other room!), make sure you've tested the recipe first. Then you know it works. You don't want to wreck your brownies or make tough-as-boots burgers! Always test first . . .

Butter and margarine
Swap for dairy-free versions, which are available in all good supermarkets. And use in exactly the same quantities. If you're shallow-frying, you can use your favorite oil, like blended olive oil or canola oil.

Cheese
We know this is the big one! So many people find it hard to abstain or reduce their dairy consumption due to cheese. We found it quite easy really. But if it makes sense in a recipe, such as in a béchamel, we will use plant-based cheese, which is available everywhere now. Check out store-bought brands and test different options: shredded, melty, and spreadable.

Try the cheese before you add it to your dish—don't ruin a dish using a bad-tasting brand! Also check out nutritional yeast (see page 141), which is an easy way to add a cheesy flavor to plant-based cooking. Get experimenting to find what's best for you.

Cream

There are many dairy-free versions. Grab yourself a tub of soy, almond, or oat cream. You can also blitz up your own cashew cream with a high-powered blender (see page 139). And if you're looking for whipped cream, there are a few brands available (look in natural foods stores) or improvise by using the thick layer from the top of a can of chilled coconut milk.

Eggs for baking

There are so many alternatives now that you can use to perform the job of an egg. Binding when baking can be achieved using swap-ins: flaxseeds, banana, apple sauce, fruit purée, dairy-free yogurt, oil, or peanut butter. There are also some convincing egg replacers available in most supermarkets now. The incredible discovery of aquafaba (literally, bean juice from a can of chickpeas, which whips up exactly like egg whites) has made plant-based egg-free meringues and mousses very easy to create.

Eggs for eating

No plant-based or vegan egg is going to make a convincing fried or boiled egg, but you can make a delicious and nutritious scramble with tofu and turmeric, and create quiches, pancakes, omelets, and frittatas with ingredients like tofu or chickpea flour.

Fish

Store-bought fish replacements are fairly easy to find, from plant-based fish fillets to fish burgers, shrimp, and canned tuna. You can also make your own versions: tofu is frequently used as a replacement for fish, as it replicates the texture of cod very well—just add a little lemon, vinegar, caper brine, and nori for a fishy flavor. We've also found that wrapping tofu in nori is a great way to mimic fish skin while adding a really fishy flavor, and shredded nori sheets sprinkled over dishes are marvelous for adding extra fishiness. If you're after fish chowder, you can try mixed mushrooms (along with those fishy flavors) to create realistic fishy chunks. Also ¾-inch rounds of king oyster mushrooms make very realistic-looking scallops!

Gelatin

This animal product is what makes things set and is used in most gummy candies. It's made by boiling skin, tendons, ligaments, and/or bones. Luckily, it's another easy swap—simply use agar powder, fruit pectin, or xanthan gum instead.

Honey

To replace honey in recipes, use the same quantity of maple syrup or other sugary syrups like agave nectar or golden, rice, or date syrup.

Meat

Much work has been done by food producers and supermarkets to replicate the distinctive, rich meaty flavor so many people miss. Veggie crumbles, sausages, and burgers are widely available. If you want to make a DIY crumbles for a shepherd's pie, lasagna, or Bolognese, blend (or finely chop) hearty veggie sausages or veggie burgers. Or you can use finely ground mushrooms or cooked lentils to create your own veggie crumbles.

Ian loves chef Derek Sarno's technique of using king oyster mushrooms with BBQ sauce to make the most incredible BBQ pulled pork. Check out our YouTube videos with Derek! Or chop them, press them under heat, and then roast them to make amazing "ribs." You can also use canned young green jackfruit in spring water as a pulled pork replacement. Henry also likes using jackfruit in hoisin duck pizza and instead of roast turkey.

If you're after cuts of meat, that's a bit harder, but still possible. We make good veggie steaks out of seitan, and you can buy them, too, in some larger supermarkets. You can even get hold of plant-based versions of ribs, duck, chicken, bacon, and even "faux gras" pâté. Tofu and tempeh are other alternatives. (See pages 140–141 for more info on these popular meat replacements.) Experiment with making your own bacon with marinated slices of eggplant, pepper, tofu, or even rice paper.

Milk

Super easy this one—replace cow's milk with non-dairy milk and you're good. Test out a few different plant-based milks until you find the one that's best for you. We prefer oat milk! Some brands have a barista-friendly version, which is great for making cappuccinos. If you want buttermilk, you can add a touch of lemon juice or vinegar to your dairy-free milk to make it slightly acidic. Try out milks made from almonds, oats, cashews, soy, and hemp—or have a go at making your own. We think the unsweetened ones are best.

Pastry dough

It's really easy to find plant-based dough. Ready-to-roll pie dough is available in most supermarkets and is often made with oil instead of butter or milk. Check the label to be sure—or make your own!

Yogurt

As with milk, this is an easy swap. Replace with a plant-based yogurt, which is available in most supermarkets. If you are using coconut yogurt, then of course there will be a coconut taste, so make sure to take that into account when you're cooking! Soy has a more neutral flavor.

WHERE DO YOU GET YOUR PROTEIN?

This is one of the most common questions people ask us when they think about switching to a vegan diet. People are always worried that they're never going to get enough protein on a vegan diet, and that if they're vegetarian they are going to have to eat loads of eggs to compensate. But we're here to tell you, you'll be fine!

Our body needs protein to help build and repair itself. Protein is made up from combinations of 20 amino acids. Our body can make most of them itself, but there are nine that we need to get through our diet. These are called the essential amino acids.

"Complete proteins" contain all nine essential amino acids. Meat and animal products are all complete proteins. By contrast, there are only a handful of plant-based sources of protein that contain all nine amino acids, namely quinoa, buckwheat, and soy. But that doesn't mean that in order to fulfill your protein requirement you need to only eat those sources of protein. You need to get a good mix throughout the day to make sure you get all nine of the essential amino acids across everything that you eat. For example, combining bread and peanut butter gives you all nine essential amino acids. Or anytime you eat grains and beans together (such as rice and peas or chili with rice) you are getting all those amino acids together, too. So just eating a wide variety of different foods means you will get all your body needs.

Our quick protein wins

- Reduced-fat hummus with whole wheat pita or falafel.

- Granola with yogurt (try mixing in a tiny bit of protein powder), topped with fresh fruit and berries, nuts, seeds, and a dollop of peanut butter.

- An on-the-go raw protein bar.

- Make your own protein balls using nuts, seeds, and oats, as well as prunes and additional flavorings.

- A massive (normally green) smoothie packed with good veggies, a few well-selected healthful fruits, and some protein powder and peanut butter with dairy-free milk (see our green smoothie recipe on page 188).

- A high-protein daal—packed with protein and fiber in the form of lentils—and spiced to perfection. (Check out Ian's Delightful Daal from **BISH BASH BOSH!**)

"YES" SNACKS

There are two types of people in this world: those who like the occasional naughty snack, and those who are liars!

We love to snack. But when you adopt a plant-based diet, snacking is probably the thing that changes the most. If you're the kind of person who can resist the temptation of a sweet treat, then good for you. But if, like us, you find yourself craving an indulgence from time to time, you'll be pleased to know you can still snack without consuming animal products. And we're not just talking about granola bars, nuts, and fruits. You can find vegan versions of chocolate cakes, cookies, cupcakes, chips, sweets, and all that naughty stuff. You simply have to know what to look for.

Gone are the days of picking a snack off the shelf without a second thought as to what is in it. It came as a bit of a shock to us how many of our favorite brands of potato chips contain milk powder and how many candies are filled with gelatin. See page 165 for the key ingredients to look out for.

Cookies and cakes

Cookies are usually branded goods, so a quick online search will give you a list of those suitable for vegans. Home-cooked cakes are typically made with eggs, milk, or butter, so assume they're not vegan. Look for the words "plant-based," "vegan," or "free from." If you aren't sure, ask!

Cereal

Most cereals are plant-based (obviously we'll use plant-based milk). Read the label and the ingredients to find out for sure. Animal-derived ingredients that we avoid in cereals are honey and milk in chocolate-flavored cereal.

Chocolate

This gift from the gods is plant-based, until factories mix it with milk. Go for dark chocolate, 70% or higher, and learn to love the stronger flavor—we did! There are also brands that make "milk" and white chocolate that are suitable for vegans. When reading labels, look out for ingredients like whey, milk, lactose, or buttermilk (see pages 164–167 for more info). If you're a fan of Snickers, Mars, and Twix bars then—sorry!—these all contain animal products! But you can still find plant-based versions (or learn to make your own).

Crackers

Despite names that include words like "cream" or "buttery," most crackers are vegan. Check the label and avoid milk, eggs, butter, whey, or animal shortening.

Potato Chips

Potato chips are almost always plant-based—since they (should be) made from just potatoes, salt, and oil. Salt and vinegar and chile flavors are usually good to go, too. However, cheese and onion, meat, and fish flavors typically contain meat or dairy flavorings. But not always! Many chips are also made with milk powder, so check the labels.

Dips

The key ingredients to avoid in dips are cream, yogurt, milk, or cheese. The good news is that all the best dips— hummus, baba ganoush, and guacamole—are good to buy, but even better (and cheaper) to make yourself. Some off-the-shelf guac contains milk.

Doughnuts

We would avoid most brands of doughnuts, which are typically made with eggs and milk (not to mention other nasties). But if you can't resist, hunt down specialty stores for plant-based versions.

Fudge

As it's made with butter and milk, we avoid most branded fudge. It's really easy to make yourself with plant-based milks and butter.

Ice cream

Two decades ago, this would have been hard to find, but dairy-free ice cream is now available in almost every supermarket.

QUICK SNACK HACKS

- Cut an apple into 8 slices, cut out the seeds, dip 1 slice in nut butter, then into a small bowl of raisins, and eat. Repeat 7 times and you're guaranteed to be grinning from ear to ear!

- Toast a slice of whole-grain bread, spread with some nut butter and raspberry jam. Wash it down with a cup of (oat) milky tea for full effect!

- Toast a whole wheat pita, cut it into soldiers, dip it in hummus, spoon on a little vegan pesto, and eat! This is kinda like a vegan dippy egg.

- Pour some granola in a bowl, cover with ice-cold plant-based milk, and sprinkle with some berries.

Pancakes, crêpes, and waffles

Most pancakes, crêpes, or waffles you can buy will be made with eggs and milk. Ask the question of your local waffle hut, or this may be one to master in your kitchen (we have a great recipe online).

Pastries

Croissants—one of our favorites—we make ourselves, as they typically contain butter. Plant-based croissants, pain au chocolat, and cinnamon swirls can be found in specialty stores.

Popcorn

Well, it's just corn, so naturally plant-based if you choose sweet or salty. Butter popcorn, toffee popcorn, or salted caramel will all probably contain animal products, though. Experiment with your flavor toppings—nutritional yeast, chile flakes, and dried herbs are all good options.

Snack and protein bars

Often these are completely plant-based, but some might contain honey, eggs, or whey powder. Newer brands often say "vegan" on the packaging. As always, if you're not sure, check the labels.

Spreads and toppings

Peanut butter and jam are vegan—and delicious! Nutella, however, contains milk. Find a "free from" chocolate spread, ideally one that's palm-oil free—see page 161 for more on this—or make your own.

Candy

It's good that most candies aren't vegan, as it helps us to be a bit healthier! Softer candies often contain gelatin (pork or beef bones). Candy is typically animal-free where it is harder or boiled. However, do check the labels, as things like shellac, beeswax, and honey can find their way into the ingredients.

Toffee and caramel

This is typically made with cream, butter, or milk, but there are many "free from" versions to be found, so read the label.

Turkish delight

This sweet treat is naturally animal-free. Cornstarch is used as a thickener. Chances are that any you pick up on the shelves will be OK to eat but, as always, check the label!

IAN ON SNACKS

It's a bit of a stereotype, but also not wrong, that vegan snacks usually involve hummus. At the beginning of this year I was feeling a bit peckish, so I nipped downstairs, looked in the fridge and found a half-full tub of hummus, a couple of carrots, and half a box of sprouted lentils. Jackpot!

I dipped the carrot in the hummus, then in the sprouts. It came out looking a bit like an alien mad scientist. But it was pretty good.

Next, I did the same but added sesame seeds and dripped a few drops of Tabasco on it, too. It looked really weird now. Like an alien mad scientist who had dandruff and was bleeding! I sent a picture of it to a friend. She replied, "Urgh, it looks like something you'd see in a Petri dish through a microscope." I didn't mind the look of it though because it was tasty.

My point here is, be prepared. Sometimes vegan snacking is a bit weird, but always delicious. Don't be afraid to try something new.

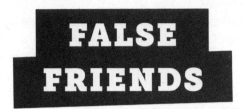

FALSE FRIENDS

It's surprising how many completely innocent-sounding food items have animal products inside them. The general rule is always check the label—see page 164 for how to read labels—but here are a few key products we've been caught out by:

Beers and wines
Isinglass (from fish bladders) is used to refine the alcohol in some wine and most real ales. Egg, gelatin, or casein (a milk protein) is often used in the production process. Most premium lagers are completely fine. See page 192 for more on booze.

Bread products
Typically, bread is just made with flour and water, but sometimes there are versions that catch you out. Brioche buns and croissants usually contain milk and/or butter and naan breads normally contain milk.

French fries
Some high-end restaurants might deep-fry these in beef drippings or goose fat. Simply ask which fat they use—vegetable or sunflower oil is fine.

Olive tapenade
Look for tapenades that do not contain anchovies.

Pasta
Fresh pasta, whether it's regular pasta shapes or filled pasta, like tortellini, is often made with eggs to retain softness. Egg noodles are obviously made with egg. Most dried pasta and spaghetti are fine, though fettuccine is usually made with egg—but check the label to be sure.

Pesto and pasta sauces
These will often contain Parmesan or other cheeses. Look for the nondairy or "free from" versions (or make your own).

Tempura or fried and battered foods
Often the batter used to make tempura, or battered things like onion rings, will contain milk or eggs.

Vegetarian sausages, veggie burgers, or ground meat substitutes
These can be deceptive, as they might contain milk or eggs. Check the label to make sure your version is plant-based.

Waxed or coated fresh produce
Often items like apples, oranges, and avocados can be coated with wax or another glazing agent that is typically made from shellac (made from the secretions of the lac bug). For oranges and avocados, you don't typically eat it as you remove the peel, but if that bothers you, ask your store for the unwaxed versions.

Worcestershire sauce
Traditional Worcestershire sauce contains anchovies, so find a plant-based version! Henderson's Relish is a great option if you are lucky enough to be in the North of England!

As always, our advice is to read the label. But cut yourself a bit of slack, too.

Don't be too hard on yourself when making decisions about the more borderline products like waxed fruit. Do it your way and you'll find it easier, and be most likely to keep eating more plant-based foods, as well as making it look effortless to those around you.

PALM OIL

This is a big one. Although technically a vegan ingredient—it's made from plants—the production of palm oil has resulted in the devastation of huge parts of the rainforest worldwide, and therefore the homes of millions of animals, birds, and insects along the way. [104]

Palm oil is single-handedly responsible for a huge amount of rainforest deforestation.

It's a really interesting topic because it brings the idea of what it means to be vegan into a broader context. There are people who argue that palm oil can't possibly be vegan, as animals are harmed in the farming of it, but most food production has an impact on wildlife and its natural habitats—even the combine harvester that gathers the wheat to make your bread . . .

Personally, we try to avoid palm oil wherever possible, but we don't chastise ourselves if we occasionally consume products that contain it. This is an opportunity for you to make your own decisions about where you stand and how far you want to take your veganism.

Whatever you decide, be aware that palm oil is in many things—from cakes and cookies to vegan spreads and some nut butters. You're already doing a great thing by eating more vegan food, so don't make it too hard for yourself. One step at a time.

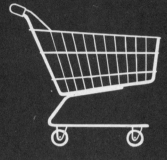

SHOPPING

THE LANGUAGE OF LABELS

When you move toward a more plant-based diet, you'll start reading the labels of food a lot more. For some people it can be one of the more off-putting things about making this lifestyle change. But stick with it and soon you will develop an encyclopedic knowledge of what products contain animal products! Then it's really easy to scan a label and make a decision in seconds.

The added benefit of this is that you will become far more aware of what you are putting in your body. Every time you check a label, you'll see if it contains any animal-derived products, but you'll also quickly notice if it contains loads of chemicals and preservatives—which does make you think twice. You may find that it's easier to stay a bit healthier with your choices when you are reading the labels of everything you eat. It also means you will be supporting businesses that are making higher quality food that's often better for the planet, too.

HOW TO READ THE LABEL

Is it an ingredient? Or is it a food that contains a combination of ingredients? If it's just a single ingredient, then you simply need to ask yourself "Did this come from an animal?" If it's a food that contains a combination of ingredients, then flip it over and read the ingredients listed on the back. Go through the following checklist—and look anything up online that you're not sure about:

1 Does it include the words "plant-based," "100% plants," "suitable for vegans," "vegan" or "vegan recipe?" If so, then it's all plants and contains no animal products. Look out for the Vegan Society's sunflower vegan trademark and the certified vegan, PETA-approved, or the Vegetarian Society vegan approved logos. Seeing these labels gives us immediate confidence that a product is vegan and that we don't need to spend ages checking the ingredients.

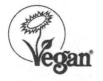 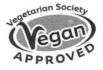

2 Does it say "suitable for vegetarians"? That's a good start, but you'll still need to check that it doesn't contain any dairy or eggs. Watch out for items that say "dairy-free," too. These often contain other animal products, such as eggs, so read the rest of the label carefully.

3 Now check the list of ingredients: do you see any animal-derived ingredients? Look for any of the obvious ones first, e.g., meat, fish, dairy, eggs, or honey. Legally, food labels must highlight common allergens—the most frequently found in nonvegan ones are eggs, milk, whey and casein—and they should also be in bold, which is helpful.

4 Now check the list below;[105] if the label lists any of these it means it is not vegan:

Albumen/albumin: this usually comes from eggs
Casein: this is a common milk protein
Collagen: made from skin, bones, and connective tissues of animals
Elastin: found in the neck ligaments and aorta of cows
Gelatin/gelatin or aspic: obtained by boiling skin, tendons, ligaments, and/or bones
Isinglass: from fish bladders
Keratin: from skin, bones, and connective tissues of animals
Lactose: a milk sugar

Lard/tallow: an animal fat
Pepsin: from the stomachs of pigs
Propolis: used by bees in the construction of hives
Royal jelly: a secretion of the honeybee
Shellac: from the bodies of insects
Vitamin D3 and cod liver oil: a fish oil
Whey: a milk by-product from making cheese

5 Many food colorings and additives are also derived from animal sources—one of the most commonly used is **E120** (also known as carmine) which is a red food coloring made from crushed beetles. Others to watch out for when traveling in the UK include:[106]
E441: gelatin—obtained by boiling skin, tendons, ligaments, and/or bones
E542: bone phosphate—made from ground up animal bones and used to keep foods moist
E901: beeswax—used as a glazing agent
E904: shellac—another glazing agent, made from the secretions of the lac bug
E910, E920, E921: L-cysteine and its derivatives—made from animal hair and feathers, and found in some breads as an improving agent
E913: lanolin—secreted by sheep and other woolly animals. While mostly used in cosmetics, it's also often used to make vitamin D3, rendering many multivitamins and fortified foods unsuitable for vegans
E966: lactitol—from lactose, which is made from milk

6 Our final (and really important) point: the label may pass all the above criteria, but also say something like "may contain milk" or "may contain eggs" or "made in a factory that handles milk and eggs." In our opinion, that's fine. We will happily eat something that has been made in a place that also handles animal products. We just want *our* food to be made without animal ingredients. But, as always, it's your call.

And that's it! Make a mental note to remember the products—or snap a photo of these pages to keep.

Soon, checking the label becomes habitual and a part of your daily routine—always check the label before you eat something new.

THE VEGAN LABEL TEST

A bag of Thai sweet chili potato chips

Ingredients: Potatoes, Vegetable Oils (Sunflower, Canola, in varying proportions), Thai Sweet Chili Seasoning, Salt, Firming Agent (Calcium Chloride), Thai Sweet Chili Seasoning contains: Sugar, Fructose, Buttermilk Powder (contains **Milk**), Dried **Soy** Sauce (**Soybeans**, **Wheat**), Tomato Powder, Onion Powder, Hydrolysed Soy Protein, Flavorings, Garlic Powder, Dried Parsley, Chili Powder, Potassium Chloride, Dried Red Peppers, Paprika Powder, Color (Paprika Extract). **Dietary information:** Suitable for Vegetarians | Contains Milk | Contains Soy | Contains Wheat | Free From Artificial Colors | Free From Artificial Preservatives | Free From MSG (Glutamate)

These do not pass the vegan label test, as these potato chips contain buttermilk powder and in bold it says "contains milk." Why they need to put milk in Thai sweet chili potato chips is another question . . .

A bag of fizzy sweets

Ingredients: Glucose Syrup, Sugar, Gelatin, Dextrose, Acid: Citric Acid, Malic Acid, Caramelized Sugar Syrup, Fruit and Plant Concentrates: Apple, Aronia, Black currant, Carrot, Elderberry, Grape, Hibiscus, Kiwi, Lemon, Mango, Orange, Passion Fruit, Safflower, Spirulina, Flavoring, Elderberry Extract. **Dietary information:** Free From Artificial Colors

Although they don't contain any allergens listed in bold, you will see that they do contain gelatin, which is found in loads of jelly candies, and is most certainly not plant-based.

A cashew sauce pasta ready meal

Ingredients: Cheesy Cashew Cream (Soy Milk [Water, **Soybeans**, Calcium, Vitamins B2, B12, D2], Water, **Wheat** Flour, **Cashews**, Sunflower Seeds, Sunflower Oil, Yeast Flakes, Onion, Dijon **Mustard** [Water, Mustard Seeds, Spirit Vinegar, Salt], Cider Vinegar, Lemon Juice, Sea Salt, Black Pepper, Sorghum Flour), Macaroni (16%) [Whole-grain Durum **Wheat** Semolina, Water], Mushroom Bacon (Cremini Mushrooms (8%), Sunflower Oil, Liquid Smoke [Water, Natural Hickory Smoke Flavor, Vinegar, Molasses, Salt], Black Pepper), Roasted Cherry Tomatoes (Cherry Tomatoes (6%), Balsamic Vinegar [Wine Vinegar, Concentrated Grape Must (Contains: **Sulphites**], Sunflower Oil), Kale (4%), Sunflower Seeds. **Dietary information:** None

✓ This one is good to go! No animal products here.

A packet of cookies

Ingredients: Wheat Flour, Sugar, Palm Oil, Canola Oil, Fat-Reduced Cocoa Powder 4.5 %, Wheat Starch, Glucose-Fructose Syrup, Leaveners (Potassium Carbonates, Ammonium Carbonates, Sodium Carbonates), Salt, Emulsifiers (Soy Lecithin, Sunflower Lecithin), Flavoring. **Dietary information:** Suitable for Vegetarians | May Contain Milk | Contains Soy | Contains Wheat

 You'll see there are no bold ingredients, so no allergens, and you can't see any animal products among the ingredients either. You'll also notice it says "suitable for vegetarians." However, it does say "may contain milk." This means that it is made in a factory that handles milk, which is why they don't print "suitable for vegans" on the packaging. Some vegans would prefer not to eat food that has been made in the same place as anything handling any kind of animal product. We tend not to worry about this. However, you'll also see that it does contain palm oil, so we'd probably give it a miss (see page 161 for more on the gray area of palm oil).

EATING PLANTS ON A BUDGET

We were on a panel on stage in front of hundreds of people, talking about sustainable food.

One of the panel claimed that eating plant-based food was a privilege that many people are not able to afford. We disagreed, but it did get us thinking.

Plant-based, vegan or veggie food is not expensive. Most of the things that people eat every day (whether they are a meat eater, veggie, or vegan) are made from plants. It's often the meat and animal products that are the expensive parts of a meal. Now, eggs are a cheap source of protein unavailable to vegans, yes, but beans and other legumes can be found incredibly cheaply, especially if you buy them in bulk. If we're talking about really, really cheap prepared meals or fast food, then yes, it might be easier to find cheap nonvegan versions. But with a bit of knowledge about how to cook, you can absolutely make healthy vegan meals on a budget.

This kind of food is not a privilege, and it can be affordable for everyone. Being vegan may even end up saving you money (see pages 76–77). Here are our top tips for eating plant-based food and keeping food costs down.

Buy ingredients

This sounds obvious, but what we mean is don't buy ready-made meals. Buy whole ingredients and cook them yourself. It's cheaper to cook from scratch and usually healthier, too, as your meals will be less processed.

Don't go shopping when you're hungry!

This doesn't just apply to your vegan supermarket shop, but any kind of food shopping! You'll make bad choices and pick up food to satisfy your immediate hunger cravings. So, avoid shopping when you are feeling peckish. Go with a full stomach (or shop online) instead.

Buy frozen

Frozen fruit and veg is usually cheaper and is often actually fresher than "fresh," as it is frozen as soon as it's picked. Look for fruits, berries, vegetables, and even herbs in the frozen aisles.

Stock up on reduced or on-sale items

Buy ingredients when they are on sale—bulk-buy plant-based milk or condiments as they have a long shelf life. Look out for fresh produce that needs to be sold that day, then freeze it until you are ready to use.

Resist "vegan," "free from," or "alternative," products

If you're looking to save money, then avoid products that are specifically "vegan" or "free from" alternatives—things like dairy-free cheese or meat-free sausages—which can be expensive. If you really want to eat them, then why not make your own? When you're starting out it can be easy to fall into the trap of buying vegan prepared meals and vegan items, but we encourage you to learn how to cook a few basic plant-based meals for yourself so you'll never be caught short—see page 202 for some of our go-to quick meal ideas.

Choose store-brand products

These can be so much cheaper than some of the big brand names. Most supermarkets also offer store-brand dairy-free products, so hunt them out; just remember to check the labels. A great way to spot the cheaper products is to look down when you are shopping—the value-priced items are often closer to your feet.

Buy in bulk

This is a really key tip—bulk-buy to get maximum savings. If you can, find a bulk-buy store; otherwise look for the bigger, cheaper bags of goods. Pantry goods will keep in your cupboards or you can freeze fresh items such as onions, carrots, and peppers.

Shop in local ethnic markets

Specialty stores can often be cheaper when buying certain goods. Whether it's spices, vegetables, tofu, noodles, dried legumes, canned tomatoes, or even peanut butter, you'll be surprised by how much you can save shopping around.

Visit your local market

Getting your fresh produce from the market can be a real money-saver. We're not talking about exclusive farmers" markets in fancy parts of town—they can be unnecessarily expensive. Find regular fruit and veg markets with low prices and be proud that you're supporting local businesses.

Eat more seasonally

Being aware of what's in season can help you make cheaper choices. Look online for what is grown in season throughout the year where you live. We absolutely love it when soil-covered new potatoes are available in abundance at the beginning of the summer. A good, herby new potato salad is the perfect accompaniment to any barbecue. We're also super stoked at the end of summer when the thorny bushes at the back of Ian's mum and dad's garden are bursting with big juicy blackberries. Perfect for pies.

Freeze fruits and veggies

Got some fruit and veg going off in the fridge? Pop it in the freezer; this saves money and reduces food waste—much better for the environment. Peel, chop, and seed as needed first, then freeze in a freezer-proof container for up to two months. We love to peel, slice, and freeze bananas to put in smoothies or to make ice cream. And we also try to batch our smoothies, using freezer bags to make ready-to-blend smoothie mixes.

Cook; don't order in

Cook as many meals at home as you can. Like anything, the more you cook, the more skilled you'll become, and find ways to make cheap and satisfying meals.

Become a creative cook

Learn to be creative in the kitchen, so you can create meals with whatever you have in the fridge. Cooking different food regularly will help you develop these skills. Mastering the art of "fridge-raid recipes" will serve you well, time and time again. The principle is simple: use what you have and create something simple but delicious. Fridge-raid roast vegetable pasta often comes to our rescue using up veggies that would have otherwise gone to waste. Here's a quick example of fridge-raid pasta:

Set the oven to 350°F. Chop **1 zucchini**, **1 bell pepper**, and **1 red onion** into chunks, throw them in a roasting pan, drizzle with a little **olive oil**, season with **salt** and **pepper** and roast for 25 minutes. Take the pan out of the oven, pour in a **can of diced tomatoes**, sprinkle with **½ tsp Italian seasoning**, season, and stir everything together to combine, return the pan to the oven for 20 minutes more. When the veggies are roasting, prep some **penne pasta** according to the package instructions. Take the roasting pan out of the oven, pour in the penne with a splash of pasta water, fold everything together, and serve.

Of course "fridge raid" isn't all about pasta—the possibilities are endless! Stir-fried whole wheat noodles, vegan omelets using chickpea flour, quick bean chili, Asian-style fried rice, tofu steak, and griddled greens, roast vegetable soups, scrambled tofu on toast and couscous salads can all be cooked super quickly and save the day when you're hungry!

Grow things
If you have the space, whether it's a small garden, yard, or just a windowsill, a great money-saver is growing stuff. You can grow fresh herbs or chiles on a window, or potatoes, zucchini, tomatoes, and all manner of healthy veg in a small backyard. This is also environmentally friendly and you know that it's all healthy, free of chemicals, and good for you.

Use dried beans
Cans of beans (e.g., chickpeas) are convenient, but it's much cheaper, and also better tasting, if you cook your own. Dried chickpeas are best cooked by soaking overnight and then simmering for about 35–60 minutes (depending on your

recipe), so you can control the texture. And although it takes a long time, if you increase your batch size you can then freeze some, so you have some ready for future meals. Dried beans will literally last for decades. After about two years in the pantry, they will lose their moisture and need to be soaked and cooked for longer than usual. But they don't lose any of their nutritional value. [107]

Batch-cook and freeze

Batch cooking and freezing can be a money- and time-saver. Make a double, triple, or quadruple batch of chili and freeze the leftovers in single portions. They'll be ready to reheat in a microwave or oven whenever you need; this is quicker than cooking and healthier than a store-bought prepared meal.

Plan your meals

Perhaps the single best way to save money is to plan your meals on a weekly basis. We spend some time on the weekend planning what we will eat over the coming days, then we write a shopping list and get everything in one weekly shop. This will help you plan ahead and keep costs down. See page 230 for more on meal planning.

We live in a houseshare with Henry's fiancée, EmJ, and our pal Anna (hey, Anna!). We're all vegan, we all love food, and we're all very keen cooks. We also like to save money where and when we can. Like many other people in houseshares, we have a house WhatsApp group. On days when we haven't planned ahead, our group usually becomes active at around 5 p.m. when we start saying things like "GANG! What's for dinner?," "I fancy cooking, who's in?" and "EmJ, you gonna make a hotpot tonight then or what?" Once we've negotiated what we're eating and who's cooking, one of us will head to the store after work to grab the ingredients we need. We split the bill so no one is left out of pocket. If you live with people who aren't vegan, that's OK! You could still use this system on the days you want to cook. In fact, the more you use this simple system, the more vegan food your housemates will end up eating, so it's a win-win all round!

Leftovers for lunch
A great hack (and one that we incorporate into our daily lives) is to have leftovers for lunch. Cook a big meal like a curry, chili, or pasta dish, and have your leftovers for lunch the next day, with a little helping of greens or salad. Hey presto, you've got two meals for the price of one (slightly bigger) meal.

Invest in a basic cookware set (if you don't have one)
Some people don't cook because they don't have the right equipment. While it can be expensive, it doesn't have to be. At the time of writing you can buy a basic starter set, including pans, knives, a sheet pan, wooden spoons, scissors, and cutlery for the price of a couple of takeout meals—and they'll last a lot longer! Get the right tools to cook, and you'll find it easier to cook and save money.

Here's our essential kit list:

- sheet pans and baking sheets
- cutting boards
- colander
- fine grater or Microplane
- foil
- food processor (and/or stick blender)
- frying pan
- garlic press
- grater
- grill pan
- heatproof bowl
- kitchen timer
- knives—at least three good-quality ones, plus a sharpening steel
- measuring cups
- measuring spoons
- mixing bowls
- oven-to-table serving dishes
- rolling pin
- saucepans—including some good nonstick ones—with tight-fitting lids
- sieve
- slotted spoon
- spatula
- storage containers (we prefer glass)
- tofu press
- tongs
- vegetable peeler
- kitchen scale
- whisk
- wooden spoons

GROCERY SHOPPING

WITH HENRY AND IAN

Our first few trips around the supermarket as vegans were crazy. We're sure the security guards were watching us as we walked up and down the same aisles, picking things up, putting them down again, and repeatedly checking our phones. At least once we gave up and bought a falafel wrap instead!

The minute you start to shop for plant-based or vegan foods, your supermarket looks very different. There are tens of thousands of items in a typical supermarket . . . that's a lot of labels to check! To navigate this many products, you need some strategies. Here goes . . .

TOP TIPS

1. Take your phone with you so you can look up ingredients you're not sure about.
2. Take a list. Be prepared and know what you're shopping for.
3. Always check the label . . . we can't say this too many times. (See page 164.)
4. Consider online shopping instead—plan for the week and get everything delivered.

IN THE SUPERMARKET

1 First up, it's handy to know that the outside aisles tend to have the fresher products, as it's quicker to get them to the shelves from the loading bays. So, around the outside we'll fill up on a load of fresh fruit and veg. Things like bananas, apples, oranges, peppers, tomatoes, lettuce, spinach, eggplant, zucchini, garlic, and onions. We'll also grab some fresh herbs and fresh bread (checking first that the bread isn't covered in cheese!).

2 Next, we'll head to the dried goods and can aisles to grab some pasta, rice, and canned tomatoes. We'll get some other canned and jarred vegetables, too—we love roasted red peppers in oil, sun-dried tomatoes, and corn, plus canned or dried beans for protein, including black beans, kidney beans, and chickpeas for making hummus. And we'll pick up some nuts and flaxseeds when we see them, to add healthy fats and omega-3 fats to smoothies and granola.

3 Now, we want to add some extra flavor, so we're going to head to the spice aisle—for a quick hit we'll get salt, pepper, paprika, chile flakes, cumin, ground cinnamon, and some Italian seasoning. While we're here, we'll pick up some olive oil, sesame oil, and balsamic vinegar, so we've got the ingredients for a quick dressing for any salad.

4 Next up, we'll grab a couple of tasty pasta or curry sauces in case we need an instant meal. We'll have a look at some labels to make sure they don't contain animal products (check our guide on page 164).

5   This is a strong-looking cart right now! People are looking at us and wondering just why we are so healthy. Already we're in a great place and have enough to eat for several days, but let's continue.

6   We're more than halfway through now, so we're on to the dairy-free dairy. We'll pick up a couple of cartons of oat milk (our favorite) and some coconut yogurt. We might also hunt down some dairy-free cheese. If we find a new brand we've not tried before, we'll see how we like it!

7   Now we're in the frozen aisle where we'll grab berries (which are perfect for smoothies) and veggie sausages. And our favorite brand of burger. There's the option of some dairy-free ice cream (some great ones are available now) so we can treat ourselves!

8   Now, and only now, are we going to head to the "free from" or vegan aisle. We've got most of what we need already (and more cheaply than buying ready-made "vegan" versions) but we'll pick up a jar of dairy-free pesto and maybe a little box of brownies. Delicious!

9   The cart is packed with fruits, veggies, and simple baked goods. We've a few ready-to-go sauces and some meat alternatives for those times we need a quick meal, but overall our cart is full of freshness, goodness, and color. Now we can check out and get on with living vegan!

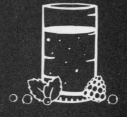

DRINKS

A NICE CUP OF TEA

People often ask us what the hardest thing is about eating all plants. We tell them it's having to wake up at 5 a.m. to milk the almonds.

Just kidding! If you rely on your caffeine fix, the good news is that tea, coffee, and most hot drinks are all plant-based. There's really only one thing to consider when it comes to most hot drinks, and that's milk. Plant-based milks are readily available in all supermarkets and there are plenty of varieties.

Despite what some people claim, plant-based milk is categorically as good as (if not better than) milk from cows (see page 85). Yes, you need to experiment to find your favorite, and if you're making lattes you'll want to get a specialty option that froths to perfection, but ultimately you'll find the flavor of a good plant-based milk can be truly delightful, and cow's milk can start to taste a little, well, icky.

Coffee, espressos, lattes, flat whites, frappuccinos, ventis, etc.

If you are a no-milk coffee kind of person, then you're in luck! Coffee is all plants (it's just coffee beans and water) so you have nothing to worry about. You can carry on drinking your espressos, Americanos, filter coffee, or instant coffee (what the French call *pipi de chat*) in full confidence that it's plant-based. Try to get Fair Trade coffees if you can. These promote positive conditions among coffee bean farmers.

If you prefer a milkier coffee, then you'll want to move to a plant-based milk. Despite what you might think, most coffee shops will happily accommodate you. It would have been much harder to do this 5 or 10 years ago, but nowadays there are so many options.

If we have a free choice of plant-based milks, we usually choose **oat milk**. It has the lowest environmental impact—meaning it takes the least amount of water and energy to make.[108] It's also delicious, has a fairly simple taste, and the best brands have barista versions available that make incredibly frothy coffees. **Soy milk** is another good choice. It has a nice consistency and quite a simple, sweet flavor.

Almond milk is very tasty—and makes great lattes if done right. You may also want to try out **coconut milk** as an option—it does have a fairly strong coconut flavor.

Try them all and see which you like best!

Teas, infusions, and nearly all leaves in hot water

The beauty of tea is that it's basically just leaves flavoring water, so like coffee, it's naturally plant-based. If you're British, then it's fairly likely you'll like a bit of milk with your cuppa. Oat is good, soy is good, too (and has a sweetness that works well in tea), and you can also find super-tasty cashew milk. Almond doesn't quite work, as it doesn't mix in so well. Experiment to find your favorite. Like with coffee, nearly every good café should now have dairy-free versions available.

If you're drinking tea without milk (like the rest of civilization) then whatever tea, infusion, or steep you are drinking, it is likely to be all plants. But do watch out for anything that contains honey. Instead of honey, lemon, and ginger, choose lemon and ginger (and if you do want the sweetness, use maple syrup or regular cane sugar—although see page 138 for more on sugar's vegan credentials).

Hot chocolate

Most drinking chocolate is not plant-based, as it contains milk. Even though it's super easy to make hot chocolate plant-based, you aren't likely to find it in a regular coffee shop. Likewise, if you like cream or marshmallows on the top, you're going to struggle. While there are a couple of brands of whipped cream and marshmallows that are plant-based, they are few and far between.

To make your own vegan hot chocolate, pour a cup of your choice of **plant-based milk** into a small saucepan, and heat gently until simmering, but not boiling. Add a few blocks of **high-quality dark chocolate**, and stir until melted. Taste, and add a little **sugar** if you need to.

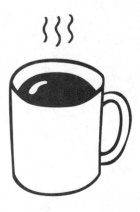

HENRY SPILLS THE TEA

I drink a lot of coffee. We work really hard at **BOSH!** and I've been known to have as many as five coffees some days. I know I should drink less, but it's so damn good to help me power through the day!

My drink of choice is either an espresso or an oat milk latte. Oat milk is one of the most environmentally friendly plant-based milks (as it uses less water in its production than, say, almonds),[109] but I'll use whatever is available. A latte is a good way to get calcium and B_{12} into your day, too.

EmJ, however, goes for tea. She drinks about five cups a day, which is probably standard for most people in Britain! She's a proper Midlands lass, and getting plant-based tea right was very, very important to her.

She experimented with all the plant-based milks, then settled on oat milk, although soy milk and cashew milk work well, too. Almond milk, on the other hand, can split and make the tea taste a bit nutty. And you would have to be bonkers to have coconut milk with tea!

SMOOTHIES AND JUICES

A green smoothie a day keeps the doctor away. We are asked all the time about how to get nutrition right on a vegan diet. Our top tip, as well as popping a multivitamin every day, is to start your morning with a big smoothie, packed with greens and healthy nutrients.

Rhonda Patrick (a PhD in human physiologist) combines apple, avocado, banana, blueberries, carrots, chard, kale, flaxseeds, spinach, and tomatoes to create a multivitamin super drink packed with thiamine, folate, magnesium, manganese, potassium, and copper, and is a good source of dietary fiber and vitamins A, C, and K. You can YouTube "Rhonda Patrick's Micronutrient Smoothie" for more info.

We love it so much that we made our own version! This smoothie lights you up like a Christmas tree.

Put **¼ cup kale**, **¼ cup spinach**, **¼ cup chard**, **8 blueberries** and **¼ cup water** into a blender and whizz for 1–2 minutes until you have a smooth paste. Scoop the flesh of **½ avocado** into the blender. Add **½ banana**, **½ apple**, **2 cherry tomatoes**, **1 tbsp peanut butter**, and a generous **¾ cup water**. Blitz until you have a thick and creamy smoothie (if you prefer it a little thinner, add a bit more water). Drink and feel healthier all day long.

Even if you buy a green smoothie in a shop, it's still good to get lots of green into your body. Just make sure your store-bought smoothie doesn't contain milk or honey—always ask before you order it. They can simply replace the milk with plant-based milk.

A little scoop of protein powder can be a great way to refuel after a workout; often it will be added to smoothies by default. Always check that the protein powder they've used is plant-based. Most protein powders are made from whey, which is derived from milk, and is definitely not plant-based. Check it's made from something like hemp, pea, or sunflower protein instead.

Fresh fruit juices don't tend to have anything added that isn't plants. Perhaps there might be someone somewhere who would put honey in a juice, but generally, when buying a juice from a shop, you're all good.

If you're buying cartons of orange, apple, or any other juice, then choose 100% juice if you can, which should be pure fruit. However, some niche and cheaper juices may contain fish gelatin or vitamin D3 (which may be derived from sheep's wool) to give the drink a nutrient boost. If in doubt, read the label.

WATER

The best drink of all is water! Water is vital for good health generally, but if you're eating more fruit and veg, you'll be upping your fiber intake, so ensure that you're adequately hydrated, too.

If you drink about eight glasses or 64 ounces of water each day, you'll be sorted. If one or two of those glasses ends up being a fizzy drink, juice, or coffee, then you'll still be fine. But aim to get at least that amount into your body every day.

If you're one of those people who claims they don't like the taste of water, then, well, you need to get over yourself! You are a human being who is in control of what you do, and you can decide to start liking water! Once you appreciate its healing properties and clean taste, you can finally move into a grown-up phase of your life where you move away from sugary drinks—and save money, too!

TAP?

Tap water is free, safe, and available to everyone. You can buy really cheap water filter pitchers for your fridge that remove some of the impurities. We've had one since we first moved to London. Countryside water is often a lot cleaner-tasting than city water . . .

HOW TO CARRY WATER

Perhaps one of the biggest marketing success stories in recent times is bottled water. Before, the idea of buying a bottle of water (which is freely available) would have seemed ridiculous. Today, plastic bottles are ubiquitous in modern society, so much so that the waste has contributed to an international cry to reduce single-use plastic. In fact, in 2018, the phrase "single-use" was Collins Dictionary's word of the year.

So, let's all follow the lead of our zero waste buddies, environmental activists Lauren Singer and Venetia Falconer, and get a reusable bottle to carry and refill as needed.

BOOZE

When Henry was 21, traveling around Australia, he remembers drinking bucketloads of "goon." That's the affectionate term for super-cheap wine served in boxes, often drunk straight out of the silver bag by long-haired backpackers (of which Henry was one). He remembers the disgust he felt the moment he discovered these cheap wines were frequently made with eggs and fish gills. Who would put that into wine?

Fast-forward to when we both started living plant-based, and discovered that almost exactly the same is true of many alcoholic beverages! A shocking number of beers are filtered with isinglass (derived from fish). And there are many varieties of wine that contain (or are processed with) nonvegan ingredients, including gelatin (animal protein), casein (milk protein), and albumin (egg protein).

All kinds of weird things get used in alcoholic drinks—insects, blood, bones, crabs, gelatin, honey, fish bladders . . . Luckily, these are the exception, as most alcohol and spirits are—thankfully—plant-based.

Unlike with foods, though, this isn't usually printed on the label, because it's part of the manufacturing process, rather than an ingredient. We know plenty of people who are plant-based, veggie, or vegan who don't worry about how their alcohol has been made. If you're like them, then skip ahead.

But if you'd rather be sure that your wine hasn't been filtered through fish bladders, read on, and we'll show you just how to be sure that your booze is free from animal products.

Beers and ciders

As a rule of thumb, lagers are usually plant-based and veggie-friendly, but real ales are not. Premium lagers (especially European ones) tend to be free from animals. In fact, Germany and Belgium have very strict purity laws for their beers. There are a handful of premium beers that aren't currently suitable for vegans, so do check the label. You shouldn't have trouble finding an alternative.

Real ales tend to use isinglass (fish bladders) as part of the filtration process, making them unsuitable for vegans. Since real ales are more seasonal, bar staff may be less knowledgeable about how each ale has been made. Although, in a good bar, they should look it up for you. The good news is some bigger, newer real ale companies are moving away from isinglass, so vegan versions are starting to appear on the market.

Ciders typically contain gelatin in the filtration process.
This is also changing, however, so check online to find out
the latest information. With more and more vegans, veggies,
and flexis, there's clearly an impetus for these brands to
go plant-based.

Wine, Prosecco, and Champagne

You would think that wine (which is basically just grapes)
would be plant-based. However, as with real ale, wine,
Prosecco, and Champagne are frequently filtered using
products (or finings) derived from animals. The finished
drinks don't necessarily *contain* the fish, egg, or gelatin
finings that have been used to purify them, but they have
been filtered through them.

We personally find the idea of fish bits dribbling through
our wine a bit horrible, so we look for natural wines.
Natural wine is a bit of a loose term, but it broadly means
wines that have been handmade with minimal processing,
little or no filtration (so no isinglass), and no additives or
sulphites. They are, therefore, typically organic and 100%
plant-based. The wines may not last as long, but they will, in
theory, also be better for you and better for the planet, and
the lack of sulphites may give you less of a hangover. The
good news is, more and more supermarkets and restaurants
are offering vegan-friendly wines, so don't be afraid to ask.
Alternatively, check a vegan listings site like barnivore.com or
go to an online store that specializes in them.

Liquors and spirits
The good news? Vodka is 100% plants! And so is pretty much any clear liquor or spirit that exists, including gin, tequila blanco, and schnapps. So clear spirits are a resounding yes, unless they contain honey. This is also the case for a couple of rums and bourbons that are flavored with honey. In general, though, bourbon, Scotch, Irish whiskey, Aperol, and rum are all naturally plant-based.

Drinks like Baileys and Advocaat are not vegan, although you can now buy dairy-free versions of Baileys, and Kahlúa is vegan! If in doubt, though, check on a vegan directory like barnivore.com.

Pre-mixed drinks
We don't recommend you drink cans of pre-mixed cocktails (we think pre-mixed rum and ginger should be a criminal offense), but if you're partial to these drinks, then check the labels. Most will be plant-based, but some may use unnecessary milk products or honey.

Cocktails
Most cocktails are vegan if they use the spirits above. You can sip most varieties of caipirinha, mojito, margarita, martini, old-fashioned, espresso martini, Jägerbomb, Moscow mule, daiquiri, Singapore sling, or cosmopolitan without having to worry about animal products.

There are a few cocktails you should definitely avoid—or request dairy- and egg-free versions. These include whiskey sours, Amaretto sours, or any other sour cocktail that uses egg white to thicken the drink. You can simply have the same drink without the egg white (or use aquafaba instead—see page 146)—an easy adjustment to make.

If you're in a quality establishment, then you can, of course, ask your bartender. He or she should be knowledgeable enough to guide you toward a plant-based cocktail.

White Russians, or any version of this milky cocktail, are often not suitable as they're made with cow's milk. You may be able to ask for a plant-based alternative.

Chambord / black raspberry liqueur—a bit of a surprising one, but this is sweetened with honey. In our younger pre-vegan days, we had a lot of parties (we even had a hot tub on the roof, though that's another story)! One of our favorite cocktails was Prosecco mixed with a touch of Chambord (it might also have a frozen grape!). Imagine our horror when we realized Chambord was not vegan. We stopped drinking it immediately, and now that we're a bit older and wiser, we've cut down on the hot tub parties, too!

Bloody Mary—this classic cocktail is not, by default, plant-based or even vegetarian. It contains Worcestershire sauce, made with crushed anchovies. Ask them to hold the Worcestershire sauce, or use a vegan alternative.

Soft drinks and mixers

Most soft drinks are vegan-friendly, so nearly all brands are suitable. They should provide full dietary information on the Nutrition Facts part of the label, so do check if you're not sure.

However, drinks that are bright orange may use finings derived from fish gelatin to stabilize the unnatural-looking orange color.

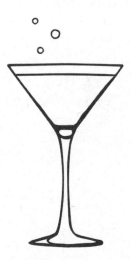

COOKING

COOKING WITH PLANTS

For us, adopting a vegan diet felt like a brain reset. We'd always been passionate about cooking, and had an arsenal of signature dishes.

When we decided to go plant-based, all this disappeared, like a tablecloth whipped out from under the plates. Suddenly, all our cooking experience was redundant. We thought none of our favorite dishes would work any longer. But luckily, we were wrong.

We were particularly worried about the staple dishes we'd mastered. Spaghetti Bolognese was a go-to dinner we'd eat at least once a fortnight. A dish we had to veganize immediately! The simple solution was substituting minced mushrooms for the ground beef in the sauce.

We used to eat fish and chips as if they were going out of fashion—so we swapped cod for firm tofu, which we flavored with lemon juice, caper brine, and nori. We battered it, fried it, and served it with double-cooked chips and it was to die for. "Tofish" and chips is now served in forward-thinking fish and chip shops everywhere. Even super-simple dishes like beans and cheese on toast with a mug of tea had to be rethought. We had to find good vegan butter, cheese, and milk to replace the dairy versions. Needless to say, after a fair bit of trial and error, beans and cheese on toast is as good as it ever was!

Nearly all your favorite dishes can be cooked with plants. That's the contents of our first two cookbooks, which are jam-packed with our favorite recipes, all using only plants. That steak and fries you used to love? **BOSH!**ed it. The best lasagna ever? **BOSH!**ed it. A big juicy cheeseburger, dripping with oil and naughtiness? **BOSH!**ed it. Everything can be cooked vegan-style. And with our **BOSH!** cookbooks and YouTube channels it's been our mission to show you how.

Plant-based foods are packed with color, flavor, and texture, and they offer such broad potential for innovation. People used to think that veggie food was dull and boring, but it is exactly the opposite. Most of the best flavors are plants, whether they're herbs, spices, or simply delicious fruit and veg.

In the world, there are thousands of fruits and vegetables, many of which we've never even tasted. Embarking upon the journey of cooking vegan food helps you learn and experiment with flavors you never knew existed. When cooking without meat you are going to discover new ways to build and layer flavors, new tricks and techniques for working with ingredients, and ultimately you will become more skilled in the kitchen.

TOP TIPS

1. Equip yourself with knowledge. Find new sources of cooking inspiration in books, videos, or websites.

2. Experiment in the kitchen, starting with the meat- and dairy-based dishes you used to cook the most.

3. Learn quick hacks and swaps to improve your favorite dishes.

4. Use vegetables you're familiar with initially and introduce lesser-known ingredients to your repertoire over time.

5. Be patient and prepare. Burned onion will ruin your dish, unravel your hard work, and leave you feeling deflated.

6. If you're serious about killing it in the kitchen, enroll in a cooking class. Online courses can quite quickly take you from beginner to confident cook.

LEARN SOME NEW RECIPES

Most people have a couple of veggie recipes in their arsenal, so you're no doubt already well on your way, but practicing and perfecting a few vegan recipes is a great place to start, so you can show others just how tasty plants can be.

Our whole business is about giving people recipes free of charge—we set up **BOSH!** to help the world learn how to cook delicious meals. If you have any of our books (which aren't free, but are a very good value!), you'll have some inspiration for meals! But if not, you can check out our website (or any plant-based/vegan chef online) to find recipes you like.

To get you started, here are a few ideas for recipes to try, while you get used to cooking more plants.

BIG BREAKFASTS

An English Fry-Up or a Tofu Scramble on Toast. It's actually very easy to **BOSH!** a big breakfast. Simply sub out the sausages for veggie sausages, leave out the bacon, and get a good recipe for tofu scramble. You can cook one of these with ease and impress any hardened meat eater.

A really easy granola recipe. Granola can be assembled from ingredients you have in your cupboards—include lots of nuts and seeds for extra nutrients. It's perfect for a quick breakfast. Make it super tasty by serving with coconut yogurt, berries, and a sprinkle of flaxseeds.

A good green smoothie recipe. It's important to get your nutrients on a flexitarian, vegetarian, or vegan diet, and starting your day with a big shot of green is a really helpful, healthful shortcut. Make sure yours is packed with spinach and/or kale. We like to throw in some flaxseeds, too. If you are keen to focus on protein, then add some hemp or pea protein, as well as a banana, avocado, and some plant-based milk. Find the recipe that works for you or see page 188 for how we get our daily dose of green. Get used to making one on a regular basis and you will instantly notice an improvement in how you feel.

LUSCIOUS LUNCHES

Tofu. Our most popular recipe is crispy chili tofu, but anything involving hot griddled, baked, or shallow-fried tofu makes a perfect lunch. Learn how to press and flavor tofu well to ensure you have enough protein. We also like scrambled tofu. This is a recipe using both firm and silken tofu (we playfully named this the "two tofu technique"), which makes a brilliant brunch—and we are BIG fans of brunch.

Finely slice **2 scallions**, grate **1 garlic clove**, blend a **block of silken tofu** and press a **block of firm tofu**. Warm **1 tbsp dairy-free butter** in a frying pan over a medium-low heat, add the scallions and garlic and stir for 1 minute. Add **¼ tsp turmeric** and **1 tsp black salt** to the pan and stir them into the oil. The black salt, also known as *kala namak*, has an incredibly sulfurous odor, which mimics egg perfectly. The turmeric provides a lovely sunny color. Pour the silken tofu into the pan and stir until it's taken on the color of the turmeric. Crumble the firm tofu into the pan and gently fold until warmed through. Serve the scrambled tofu on toast, seasoned with black pepper and garnished with chives. This dish is bursting with flavor, texture, protein, and most of all, WOW factor. You'll love it.

A really good sandwich! One of our favorites is our version of a BLT, where we use strips of tofu instead of bacon (or you can find plant-based bacon in specialty stores).

Here are a few delicious sandwich ideas that will keep you going:

- chickpea tuna
- tofish fingers and minted garden peas
- BBQ tofu steak
- pulled BBQ king oyster mushroom
- vegan ham and cheese salad
- tofu egg mayo and lettuce
- roasted turkey jackfruit and stuffing
- vegan sausage and fried onions

Cheese toasties. We don't crave cheese as much as we used to, but we LOVE a cheese toastie! While they may not get quite as melty as dairy cheese, they do the job, and we like to pimp ours out with a little bit of Indian brinjal pickle. Dairy-free cheeses can be found all over (go for a melty one) or you can also create your own by blending cashews.

Brinjal pickle is easy to find in big supermarkets and there are loads of pickle and chutney recipes out there. Here's a super-simple onion pickle recipe to start you off:

Peel **1 garlic clove**, cut it in half and put it in a bowl. Add **½ tsp sugar**, **½ tsp salt** and a scant **½ cup distilled white vinegar** and stir to dissolve. Peel and finely slice **1 medium red onion** and put the slices in a colander over the sink. Pour boiling water over the slices. Drain and add to the bowl. Stir to mix and leave to rest for 10 minutes.

More than just falafel wraps

In today's busy world, sometimes we need to grab something quick to eat as we head from one thing to the next. You'll get used to knowing what to look for, but it's helpful to do a bit of research in advance to find the most veggie-friendly restaurants near you. Trial and error are your friends: wander into sandwich shops and have a look around; make a mental note of places that have lots of options and places that don't.

Do bear in mind that sandwich shops may not have ingredients listed in the same way as supermarket products. The laws are different for listing ingredients in freshly prepared sandwiches; you may need to ask to be sure.

In the bad old days, plant-based food was typically just a falafel wrap. Not that we have anything against a falafel wrap, of course. Now, eateries are constantly innovating and adding to their range of veggie foods. Ask the staff, and you can find options like sushi, Thai hotpots, soups, cookies, dairy-free baguettes, and even plant-based Thanksgiving-leftover sandwiches. If there are no meat-free options in your local sandwich bar, then they need to move with the times! But don't worry, because there's always a backup plan . . .

Get a supermarket picnic! Find your nearest local convenience store or corner shop and grab a few "picky bits." Crudités (carrots, peppers, tomatoes) and hummus is a wonderful lunchtime snack—and super healthy. Every single supermarket, no matter how small, should have a selection of hummuses. You may find falafel or potato chips or a handful of fruit and nuts. It may seem basic, but grabbing a few raw snacks is actually a great way to eat a healthy lunch when there are no convenience options available.

SIDES AND SHARERS

Cauliflower Buffalo wings. This recipe from our first book is our favorite party snack and shows how easy it is to create flavor using just plants. They are decadent and indulgent, but still healthy-ish.

Cashew cheese. This recipe works well as a simple herby cream cheese to spread on crackers—and also for dipping cauliflower Buffalo wings! Use less water for a firmer consistency:

Tip **1½ cups well-soaked cashews** and **2 tbsp water** into a blender and blitz until totally smooth. Add another **2 tbsp water, 1 tsp salt, 2 tbsp coconut oil, 1 tbsp nutritional yeast**, the juice of **1 lemon** and **1 garlic clove** (peeled). Blitz until totally smooth. Transfer the mixture to a serving bowl, add a small handful of finely chopped **fresh parsley leaves** and **6–8 finely chopped chives**. Fold into the mixture with a spoon, cover the bowl, and refrigerate until set.

Other sharing ideas. Food is best enjoyed with friends. Here are a few ideas for recipes that feed a crowd easily. You can find these recipes online or in our books. They're making us hungry just thinking about them!

- tapas
- potato nachos with vegan sour cream, salsa, and guacamole
- crispy oyster mushroom chicken wings with dips
- tacos, all the vegan tacos
- mock duck hoisin pancakes
- crudités and hummus
- seitan chicken with BBQ sauce
- pizza
- bhaji bites with spiced tomato chutney and raita
- falafel and baba ganoush
- vegan sushi

DECADENT DINNERS

Chili sin carne. Chili is one of the easiest dishes to make taste incredible, while also the one that will surprise a meat eater the most. You can make yours with minced mushrooms, store-bought vegan crumbles, or even blended-up veggie burgers or sausages. Try putting lentils in there for a little extra bite.

Lasagna. It's simple to make a good plant-based lasagna. You'll typically make a vegetable lasagna with a vegan béchamel (you'll be using "magic dust" aka nutritional yeast for this). Our favorite is our classic lasagna from **BISH BASH BOSH!**, but we also created the World's Best Pesto Lasagna, which is in our first book and on BOSH.TV. Try a few different recipes until you find your favorite—or why not **BOSH!** your own!

Spaghetti Bolognese. This was one of our favorite dishes when we were meat eaters and is a great weekend lunch, along with a bit of green salad. We often make ours with mushrooms instead of vegan crumbles, but you can also make crumbles by mashing up veggie sausages, or just buy plant-based crumbles in any good supermarket. For a truly pimped-out dish, try using good-quality vegan burgers shredded up into crumbles!

Sausage hotpot stew. This is incredibly easy to put together—just canned tomatoes, veggies, and veggie sausages will do the trick—and it goes well with a little rice or bread.

DESSERTS

Minty chocolate mousse. This easy chocolatey mousse will leave your guests wanting more:

Slowly melt **3 oz dark chocolate** in a bowl over a pan of hot water. Take the bowl off the heat and set to one side. Use a stand mixer to whip the liquid from a **14 oz can chickpeas** (aquafaba, about ½ cup) into a thick cream (stiff peaks need to form when the paddle is pulled up). Add the melted chocolate, **2½ tbsp sugar**, **1 tsp peppermint extract**, and a **pinch of salt** to the bowl and gently fold together with a wooden spoon. Spoon the mixture into serving glasses, cover, and chill overnight. Grate **½ oz dark chocolate** over the glasses, garnish with mint leaves, and serve.

Chocolate cake! Perfect for a birthday, a celebration, or Easter, a good chocolate cake should be in everyone's repertoire. We've had over 4 million views of our Ultimate Chocolate Cake, which is so indulgent and gooey it will make your mouth water just watching the video.

Cheesecake. You might be surprised to learn that you can make it without dairy. We created a wonderful New York–style strawberry cheesecake, which you'll find in **BISH BASH BOSH!**.

Ready-in-minutes chocolate chip cookies. You can't go wrong with a warm-from-the-oven cookie! They're also simple to customize. Find a recipe and go for it! Make sure yours are crunchy-on-the-outside, gooey-on-the-inside.

GREENS AND SALADS

An incredible salad dressing. Salads are easy, and you have so much flexibility with what you put in them. One of the best ways to make a salad sing is to make a lightning-quick dressing. Our go-to dressing is super simple:

Add **3 tbsp extra-virgin olive oil**, **1 tbsp balsamic vinegar**, and a pinch of **salt** and **pepper** to a sealable container and shake vigorously until everything is well mixed. That's it! Splash that over your salad and you'll be on to a winner.

A powerful and well-dressed lentil salad. This is ideal when you are looking for a protein and nutrient kick. We used to avoid lentils because we thought they were *way* too vegan. How wrong we were! Make lentils taste incredible by combining them with heaps of roast vegetables. Here's a quick and devilishly tasty dressing to make your lentils even better:

Add **3 tbsp olive oil**, **1 tsp Dijon mustard**, the **juice of ½ lemon**, and **1 tsp pomegranate molasses** (available in most big supermarkets now) to a sealable container and shake to combine. Drizzle this dressing over your lentil salad or toss the lentils in the dressing to combine.

Homemade pesto salad. Often salads are served with cheese, but a good homemade pesto achieves the same effect as cheeses like feta or Parmesan, but with pine nuts, almonds, or miso. Learn how to make an incredible dairy-free pesto, and you can quickly rustle up a wonderful salad or pasta dish:

Put **¾ cup pine nuts** (lightly toasted), **2 cups basil leaves**, **1 small garlic clove**, peeled and chopped, the **juice of 1 small lemon**, **2 tsp nutritional yeast**, a scant **½ cup extra-virgin olive oil**, **salt** and **pepper** in a blender and blitz until you have textured pesto. Drizzle it over salad, stir it into pasta, spread it on toast, or dollop it in Italian soup. You've now got a solid pesto recipe that will serve you forever.

COOKING AND EATING BY CUISINE

Different cuisines lean on different ingredients, and some are easier to make plant-based than others. So when it comes to eating out or adapting some of your favorite recipes to cook at home, it can be helpful to think about the common ingredients used in some of your favorite meals.

INDIAN

Indian food is easy to make veggie; in fact there are many parts of India that are naturally vegetarian or even vegan. Look for curries without paneer (cheese) or yogurt, cream, or butter (ghee), which are often used to add creaminess. Be specific about ghee—if you're eating out, check that they don't use it to cook the curries or breads. You can use coconut oil at home—it has the same silky texture as ghee. Naan breads are typically made with milk, so choose roti or chapati instead. Poppadoms and pickles are generally good to go—but avoid any raita dips that are made with yogurt!

When Henry went backpacking around the world, he was inspired by the contrasting flavors of Indian and Nepali curries. When he returned, he learned to cook curry (Jamie Oliver's was the first curry recipe Henry ever cooked)! Curries are wonderful; the combinations of spices mean you can layer up the flavors. Also, our discovery of jackfruit was a total game changer, and led to all number of delicious dishes like the biryani from **BISH BASH BOSH!**.

PIZZA

Pizza is easy to customize so perfect for eating out on a plant-based diet. Ask for a veggie pizza without cheese or opt for vegan cheese. Lots of restaurants will have the choice of dairy-free cheese or even a vegan pizza on the menu now. In an authentic Italian pizzeria, try a marinara pizza, which has a garlic-tomato sauce, and is naturally plant-based. If you're eating in a more American-style pizza joint (the kind that makes fluffy pizza dough), then check that the dough is dairy-free. Some places put milk in their dough.

When we make pizzas, we like to do so with friends! We always make extra dough (so we can freeze some for another time) and make an easy tomato sauce base by whizzing up tomato puree, garlic, basil, and a touch of red wine vinegar in a blender. Then we'll set out lots of bowls of pizza toppings and everyone creates their own pizzas.

BRUNCH

In a typical brunch spot, you can normally rustle up a plant-based option easily. Avocado on toast is an obvious choice, although it sometimes comes with egg or salmon so simply ask them to remove it. If they offer a full English, Irish, or American breakfast (basically all the same thing), then you can make that veg-friendly; get them to hold the bacon, eggs, and sausage, and design your own breakfast consisting of things like fried mushrooms, tomatoes, beans, toast, and, if you're lucky, a bit of spinach or avocado. And if there's oatmeal, overnight oats, or granola on the menu, ask if they can do a plant-based version of those; most discerning restaurants should carry plant-based alternatives.

And we love brunch at home! Scrambled egg (made from tofu) is Ian's favorite, then we layer on all the fried goodness—or roasted if we're feeling lazy. Henry likes brown sauce (HP). Ian likes red sauce (surely that's called ketchup?). The toast has got to be high-grade sourdough bread, and then we'll prep ourselves for a 30-minute sit-down afterwards, to let the food digest!

ITALIAN

Italian food can be variable, as it's often centered on meat, fish, and cheese. Pizza is often a good choice (see page 213 for our recommendations there), or you can opt for a simple pasta dish. A pasta arrabbiata or marinara is typically

nt-based, but be sure the pasta doesn't contain eggs.
e of our easiest, tastiest dishes is Easy Peasy Pasta.
nply pop a load of veggies, very roughly chopped, into a
king dish and bake in a 350°F oven for 30–40 minutes.
x it all with a spoon and you have an instant pasta sauce.
uschetta is an easy plant-based recipe, too, and salads are
viously great—combine with fries if nothing else will do!
me places may even create a risotto just for you if you ask
em nicely.

MIDDLE EASTERN

e of the finest cuisines for vegans, veggies, and flexis is
ddle Eastern. This catch-all category covers cuisines like
rkish, Israeli, and Lebanese. There are plenty of animal-
e mezze options to choose from, including falafel, baba
noush, hummus, tabbouleh, dolmades, and flatbreads.
ese cuisines use less milk than we do in the West, so you'll
d many more vegan-friendly options.

FRENCH

nch food is not the most veggie-friendly cuisine, so if
u're heading to a French restaurant, then it's definitely worth
oning ahead to find out what can be done—the chefs will
preciate it and be more likely to accommodate you. If in
ubt, ask for combinations of grilled veggies, green salads
th a simple vinaigrette, French fries, or boiled potatoes.

If you're cooking at home, you can be a bit more adventurou
Bourguignon has traditionally been a very meaty affair,
but times have changed. Mushroom Bourguignon is now
extremely popular and, what's more, it's extremely deliciou

Croissants that have been made with vegetable fats rather
than dairy butter can now be found in supermarkets up an
down the country and we, as we're sure you can imagine,
over the moon about that! Crème brûlée is a dish that, on
the outside, looks as if it would be very difficult to veganize
Don't worry, crème brûlée *has* been veganized and there a
loads of recipes online. Crunchy, creamy, sweet, and vegar

THAI

Thailand is one of our favorite culinary destinations! It is
fairly easy to make Thai food plant-based, since their currie
salads, and stir-fries are typically made without any dairy, s
opt for meat- and fish-free versions and you'll be all good.
But fish sauce is commonly used in Thai foods, stocks, and
sauces. We know some people who eat plant-based but
choose not to worry about fish sauce. However, we don't
eat it, so if you prefer, ask your Thai restaurant if they can
create your dish with no fish sauce. At home, vegan fish
sauce replacements are fairly easy to find in supermarkets,
or you could use an alternative like soy sauce, a vegan
Worcestershire sauce, or brown rice miso.

CHINESE

spy duck pancakes used to be one of our favorite meals in inese restaurants. We were delighted to discover pancakes ng crispy tofu in place of the duck. You could also try py mushrooms. Chinese vegetarian stir-fries are typically e for vegans, but watch out for fish sauce. And be aware t fried rices are typically cooked with egg.

VIETNAMESE

tnamese food is dairy-free by default, but often contains at, so if you can find good vegetarian dishes, then you are od to go. Vietnamese food is often centered on noodles d soups, which can be incredibly delicious—just check that stocks are not made with meat (they often are) and that y don't contain fish sauce. A veggie noodle dish made h veggie stock is ideal. Or try a zingy salad, spring or nmer rolls and dipping sauce, or wonderful veggie (egg- e) noodles.

MEXICAN

ile they eat a lot of meat in Mexico, they also do great etables. Many of the best vegetables in the world originate m Mexico, so they've learned how to cook them to fection. No cuisine epitomizes the phrase of "eating the bow" better than Mexican and Tex-Mex food. Fajitas, burritos, chimichangas, tacos, and tostadas can all be made plant-based. Just make sure it's vegan cheese and sour crea or go without and add extra guac and salsa instead! Also, a good bean chili can be as delicious (if not more so) than the meaty versions. Be sure the tortillas do not contain lard.

BURGERS AND OTHER AMERICAN CLASSICS

The incredible advances in alternative meat burgers (Beyor Burgers, Impossible Burgers, etc.) have proven that you do have to miss out on flavor. In our opinion, any good burge joint should have perfected a plant burger alongside their meaty options, but it's worth checking online to find the b veggie-friendly burger near you. Also, check that the buns and cheese are plant-based. Often brioche buns are made with milk and butter. And obviously make sure it's dairy-fre cheese. As far as convincing meat eaters about a plant-bas diet, though, we find that American classics like burgers, chil and chicken wings are the ones that make people say, "Wow can't believe that's vegan!"

If you're making a burger patty at home, make sure there a ingredients in the mixture that will help it bind and becom malleable. We've blended cooked brown pasta, cooked Pu lentils, roasted sweet potatoes, cooked brown rice, and cooked vegan sausages to make fantastic vegan burgers. Next, play with the flavor. We like to add a good amount o

IAN'S MEATMISSION EXPERIENCE

When I was about three weeks into veganism a friend invited me to a restaurant called MEATMission. As the name suggests, it was meaty. Really meaty.

This was the first time I had visited a restaurant as a vegan. When I got there, I had a drink at the bar with my friend and his buddies, then we headed over to our table. I looked at the menu and realized that the only things I could eat were, unsurprisingly, salad and fries. Everyone placed their orders. Steak. Burger. Ribs. Wings. Then it was my turn: "I'll take an order of fries and a bowl of salad. Can you ask the chef to hold the ranch?" I couldn't believe it! This was one of the best barbecue joints in the country and I'd ordered a salad and fries? I was close to slapping a rack of ribs onto my order, but I stopped myself. I thought about *Cowspiracy* and *Earthlings* and made the conscious decision to stay strong. The food came, everyone ate, we had a few more beers, and ended up having a blast. When I got home that night, I was feeling kinda smug. I had cleared the first hurdle.

umami (the savory, "meaty" taste found in Parmesan, miso, and mushrooms) and a little smokiness to our burgers. It really helps mimic the taste of flame-grilled meat.

TEXAN BBQ / SMOKEHOUSE / BRAZILIAN GRILL

This should be fun! If you're heading out to eat somewhere like this, first of all, kudos to you for going with your (presumably meat-eating) friends to a very meat-focused restaurant. We recommend you phone ahead and let them know you are coming, and ask what vegan options they can offer. They might surprise you with their vegan-friendly selection. Be prepared to deal with a little bit of light mockery (let's not take ourselves too seriously), to watch other people eating loads of meat (maybe not your favorite thing to do), and know that you may just be ordering some salad and fries! But, you clearly chose this restaurant because your friends are more important than your eating habits, so keep that in mind if they make fun of your limited food choices!

BRITISH CLASSICS

Pubs can be quite variable in their food options, so check out the menu. If you are looking for that classic British dish, the roast dinner, then you definitely should do some research online to find the best plant-based and vegan roasts near you. Veggie roast dinners tend to sell out quite quickly, so call ahead to make sure they save one for you. And then let us know how it was and we'll try the roast out ourselves! #roastdinnerseveryday

HENRY'S FESTIVE FEASTS

Last Christmas, Henry hosted EmJ's and his entire family for Christmas dinner at **BOSH!** HQ. Even the dog came! He cooked for 12 people, and the nonvegans were good enough to eat a vegan Christmas dinner. That meant he had to impress!

He spent the whole day cooking, and served up a massive spread, including **BOSH!**'s now famous jackfruit roast dinner, a mushroom Wellington, oodles of delicious rosemary-garlic roast veggies, our perfect gravy, wonderful stuffing, and a vegan yule log for dessert. It was an impressive spread and everyone loved it!

Even EmJ's nan (who was married to a master butcher) said she enjoyed it, although she did comment that she'd never seen someone making so much of an effort in the kitchen! A compliment? Let's just say it was! The roast went down a storm and all the meat eaters enjoyed it.

BOSH! YOUR KITCHEN

We hear all the time that veggie food takes ages to cook. That's rubbish.

This way of eating can be just as quick, if not quicker—or it can take as long as you want. Since the recipes are likely to be new and may involve new ingredients, at first it can take a bit longer.

Being able to whip things up quickly and efficiently is important for many reasons: it will give you confidence, let you explore new ingredients, and help you stay on track. Most important, when you're cooking for someone else, it'll seem like eating delicious plant-based food is really easy, because you nailed it!

When we are all busy, it can be hard to find the time to cook good food. The following tips will help you be a more efficient cook.

① STREAMLINE YOUR KITCHEN

"OK," we said to each other as we looked at our kitchen after just turning vegan. "We'd better hunt through here and work out what we can and can't eat. It won't do to have fridges filled with meat anymore."

And with that we set about clearing our kitchen of all animal-derived products. We took everything out and read the label. If it was "free from," we put it back in the cupboards. If it wasn't, we sent it to a local food bank.

Now this stage is totally optional. How you treat your kitchen is a very personal thing, but we think it's a good idea to streamline your kitchen so it's easier to find things when you want them. You want to know, without having to think too hard about it, where the plant-based goodies are! How you organize your space totally depends on how you live, who you live with, and how much space you have. But even if you're sharing a kitchen with other people, all you need is to create a "my foods" zone. This zone could be a cupboard and a shelf in the fridge. Or it could be the entire kitchen!

Once you've worked out your system, empty out the cupboards, putting all the products on the table. Check the labels (see page 163), and if they're free from animals, put them back in the cupboards. If they're not, then either give them to other people to eat or send them to a food bank for someone else to enjoy.

Try to keep the system going (and get others in your house to follow it, too!) and you'll find it super easy to stay on top of it, and you'll always know where there is food that you can eat.

Disclaimer: some people you live with (parents, loved ones, etc.) might not like the idea of your separate cupboards—they might even be offended! Do your best not to get into an argument. Play it by ear to find the solution that's right for you and those you live with.

2
PLAN AHEAD OF TIME

Create a weekly meal plan and shopping list to get everything delivered in one big order. It's quicker and cheaper and avoids those painful "What's for dinner?" questions. You can do this yourself (see page 230) or check out our ready-made meal plans at BOSH.TV. Just get into the habit of thinking ahead.

IAN'S FLAVOR SAVERS

- Use a good-quality extra-virgin olive oil for dressing your salads.

- Use a splash of sesame oil along with vegetable oil when cooking Asian dishes as the flavor of sesame oil alone can be a bit overpowering.

- Taste as you cook and season to taste. Use flaky sea salt instead of table salt, as the natural properties work in harmony with food and enhance flavor. Table salt tends to mask other flavors.

- A touch of acid from lemon, lime, or vinegar can really make a dish pop.

- Cook onions slowly in warm oil. This will help eke out their natural sweetness and avoid burning.

- If you're using cilantro in a curry, finely slice the stems and add them to the pan when you add the onions—they'll add another great layer of flavor.

3

GET READY TO COOK

Before you start, empty the dishwasher and clear your sink of dirty dishes. It's so much more Zen to cook in a clean kitchen. Take the extra five minutes to clear up before you start cooking. If you clean as you go, you'll find the whole process quicker and more peaceful, as you'll have less mess to avoid.

Next, get all your cookware out. Who wants to be rummaging around to locate a colander when the pasta is done? Or scrabbling around to find a wooden spoon, only to realize it's dirty, and then burning the onions! That will only create a stressful cooking experience. Have a skim through the recipe and get your equipment and ingredients ready in advance. Also think about the different steps in the recipe so you know what's coming—you'll find it easier to cook and you'll be less likely to make mistakes.

For example, a stir-fry is quickly cooked at a high heat, so it's helpful to have all your ingredients chopped and ready before you start to cook. But sometimes it is quicker and more logical to prep as you cook, for example getting a sauce on the burner and leaving it simmering while you prepare the accompaniments.

Here are some more handy hacks to **BOSH!** your kitchen:

Hack 1: Let your oven do the work

The oven can really help make your cooking more efficient. You can **BOSH!** some veg in there and let it cook. If you're wondering what to cook, just pop some veg in the oven and throw these on some pasta. Simple!

Hack 2: Get batching!

Batch-cooking gives you the gift of time in the kitchen. There are a few different ways to batch-cook. You can make things that will last for a while, like kimchi, peanut butter, jams, and hummus, and store them in the fridge in airtight containers. You can also get into the habit of doubling the quantity of whatever you're cooking and saving half for another day. Freeze batches of curries or sauces so it's super quick to rustle up a meal when you're tight on time. You could also cook a whole week's worth of food on a Sunday or spend some time cooking enough for today and tomorrow. Stock up on storage boxes and get meal-planning—you'll be amazed how much time you save!

Hack 3: Chop extra veggies

If you've taken the time to clear the kitchen and get ready, why not prep a few extra veggies? For example, by chopping more veg than you'll need for a pasta sauce, you can make yourself a salad for the following day with little extra effort. Put half of the veg you chop, like onions, tomatoes, peppers, and the like, in an airtight container in the fridge. Create a quick dressing, add some beans, and you have an instant salad. You can also freeze chopped veg.

Hack 4: Learn how to power-up dishes

Meals don't need to take ages to put together. A "few things on a plate" approach can help you make wonderful dishes really quickly. Use toppings that you batch-made earlier in the week (like salsa, hummus, or baba ganoush) to add flavor to a simple salad or **BOSH!** bowl. A little lemon juice on top of roasted veg will add instant flavor. Balsamic glaze looks stunning when drizzled over a salad. Experiment with simple power-up toppings, fats, and acids to bring out your favorite flavors.

Hack 5: Turn up the heat

Our Ultimate Chili does best when left to simmer gently for 2 hours. However, we've also cooked it in about 5 minutes on national TV. Turning up the heat (and continually stirring) lets you cook much faster. Of course, you are going to need to work hard to keep things moving, so your onions and other ingredients don't burn, but with the right amount of oil and the right amount of stirring, you can rustle up dishes like curries, marinara sauces, stews, or chilis in half the time, at a higher heat.

Hack 6: Get more people involved!

This might sound like an obvious one, but get your friends, family, or loved ones to come and help. Get them washing, chopping, stirring, or reading out the recipe—another pair of hands will help you work faster and eat sooner!

LIFESAVER RECIPES

What's in the fridge? Know how to cook it? These little lifesaver recipes can be used with most types of vegetables and mean that you've always got something for dinner.

1. Roast vegetable soup. Prep the veg, roast them in a 350°F oven, pop in a pan, add a little vegetable stock, and blend until you get the texture you want. Serve with some bread for a mighty fine meal.

2. Stir-fries. A go-to, quick way to use up veg and fill your body full of healthy goodness. Keep a couple of bags of microwavable rice and some straight-to-wok udon noodles in your cupboard. Add those amazing familiar flavors with toasted sesame oil, sriracha, and soy sauce.

3. Instant curries. Keeping a few spices such as cumin and ground coriander in your cupboard and some onions, garlic, and ginger in your fridge will give you the base you need to rustle up a quick, simple curry.

MEAL PLANNING

Meal planning is a good way to get through the week and reduces any thinking time about what you are going to eat and when. It's also a great crash course in plant-based cooking. You'll be a master in no time!

	MON	**TUES**	**WEDS**
Breakfast			
Lunch			
Dinner			
Snacks			

PRO TIPS

Consider how much you want to cook; you might find it easier to keep some leftovers from dinner and put them into a lunchbox for the next day.

Don't worry too much about snacks. You could make some granola bars or just take some fruit to work. But there's no shame in a store-bought snack or a cheeky brownie either!

Once you know what you're planning to cook, you can **BOSH!** your shopping and make one ingredients list to last the whole week. Here's a blank meal plan to get you started.

THURS	FRI	SAT	SUN

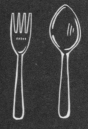

EATING OUT AND ORDERING IN

We love supporting veggie and vegan businesses, but it's actually a really good thing to order plant-based food in "normal" restaurants, too.

It's the simple rule of supply and demand. As more customers demand plant-based food, restaurants will supply more options, making it easier for everyone to order plant-based food anywhere.

Don't be afraid to chat with waiters and ask about their vegan-friendly options (see page 236 for more on this). And if you are going somewhere that you're not sure has much plant-based food, then maybe call ahead to check and let them know you're coming. The chef will be grateful and will be more likely to be able to accommodate you!

RESTAURANT & TAKEOUT TOP TIPS

1. Browse online to find good options in your area and make a list of your favorites to try. Do some research to find out which non-veggie restaurants serve good plant-based options. You'll be surprised how many have a veggie or vegan section on their menu. This means they have thought in advance about your food requirements, and the staff will immediately understand what you are asking for. Read the menus online and look for vegan (v) or plant-based (pb) options.

2. Use an app like Happy Cow (www.HappyCow.net) to help you find veg-friendly restaurants nearby.

3. Ask the staff if you're not sure; most places should have a vegan, veggie, or at least an allergen menu that will give you the information you need.

4. Design your own meals in restaurants. There are still plenty of restaurants that don't yet have clear veggie menus or well-trained staff. It's helpful—for you and them—to ask about ingredients and design your own meals. You'll want to get used to telling waiters your requirements (see page 236), and also check our guide to different cuisines (page 212).

5. It's worth phoning ahead to let them know you are coming and you'd like plant-based options. Chefs do appreciate it, and it will make it easier (and maybe less embarrassing) for you to get the food you want.

6. Search for vegan hashtags plus the name of your local area on Instagram and Twitter, such as #veganlondon or #vegansheffield (our two personal favorites!). Or look up some vegan bloggers and Instagrammers who have done all the hard work for you! Facebook groups are a handy resource for discovering local vegan eateries, too. Most towns and cities will have Facebook groups full of members who will be keen to help you out and answer any questions. Typing "Sheffield Vegans" into Facebook's search bar leads you to groups that have been set up by passionate vegan Sheffielders who are happy to share their tips. Check out your hometown!

7. Get recommendations from people, either online or face-to-face. There are vegan meet-up groups all over the country, so try going to events in your area (Vevolution in London is a great example) to hang out with like-minded people. We've found the vegan community to be very friendly and helpful, and we're sure you will, too. Of course, veggie and vegan restaurants are good places to meet people! We are lucky enough to meet fans of **BOSH!** quite often when we eat out, and we can vouch for the fact that the people eating in those places are super friendly!

8. Know what your opinion is on alcohol and whether you are looking for vegan options or not (see page 192).

9. Be prepared to discuss all the vegan questions with the guests at the table! See page 302 for some of the questions you might get asked.

HAVING FUN WITH WAITERS

Remember the good old days when you could just order food off the menu and eat it?

Well, those days are gone. Dietary requirement requests are increasing across the board and waitstaff should be fully trained in whether something is meat-free, contains nuts, gluten, or dairy, or what to do if you simply don't like mushrooms.

This is your world now: chatting with waiters. And the key to making this a positive experience is to have fun with it! Smile, feel confident, and don't be afraid to ask for what you want. You are looking for plant-based or vegan options—do they have any? It's actually quite fun finding out the different types of response to this question.

Some will have absolutely no idea what you mean and will bring you a breakfast with eggs and cheese on it when you clearly and explicitly asked for a breakfast with no eggs or cheese. You'll have to politely send that meal back (and probably not go to that restaurant again). But some will be veggie or vegan, too, and will helpfully recommend the best options on the menu. Sometimes, you'll find that the chef is plant-based, and he'll make a special dish just for you. Sometimes, though, the waiter may be rude and turn their nose up at you (try to see the funny side!). And sometimes you'll end up in a chat with the waiter about food, food choices, and sustainability.

Hack 1: Smile!
Be friendly and you'll be more likely to get a positive and helpful response. If they pull a funny face or act a little difficult, just keep going. Be clear what you are looking for and how they can help you.

Hack 2: Ask if they have a veggie or vegan menu (or an allergen menu)
The first question to ask is if they have a vegan or vegetarian menu. If they do, you are in luck! This will make your life easy, and you can order whatever you want. If they don't have one, they may have an allergen menu, which is sometimes a folder showing all the ingredients in the different menu options (they should have this by law in the UK). Check the allergens menu and find dishes that are veggie and don't contain milk, eggs, cheese, or dairy.

Hack 3: Ask if they have vegan options

If they don't have anything specifically vegan-friendly, see if there's anything that looks like it could be made plant-based. They may need to go and ask the chef—and if they do that's fine! Let them know that you're looking for vegetarian dishes, but with no eggs, no cream, no butter, no milk. We have some friends who go as far as saying they are allergic to dairy, but we think it's enough to be clear and direct.

Hack 4: If they cook a great dish—let them know!

Nothing fosters positivity more than being cheerful and grateful. If you had a delicious plate of food, tell them you loved it! Consider leaving a good review online, too, to let other people know that they are a vegan-friendly establishment.

Hack 5: If they got it wrong, let them know, too

If they send you food that isn't plant-based, politely send it back and explain why. If you had a really bad experience, then you might want to consider chatting with the manager. If that doesn't work, post an online review. Your feedback is helpful; they can improve and other people can choose whether or not to eat there.

Smile, feel
confident,
and don't be
afraid to ask
for what you
want.

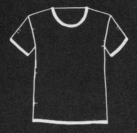

BEYOND
FOOD

We decided to cut out animal products in 2015, and to begin with it was all about the food. We quickly learned what to eat and drink and we taught ourselves to cook. Clothes were not a big focus for us at that point. We didn't buy many new clothes and we were happy with what we had.

But as time went on, we started to think more and more about the clothes we were wearing, how they had been made, and the impact they had on the world around us.

We started to question the provenance of other products we used in our day-to-day lives, too, and we tried to make choices that were more in line with our new way of thinking.

Everyone knows fur is bad, and of course we supported the brands that were moving away from it. But it got us thinking about the difference between fur and leather. Is one better than the other? What about wool, feathers, and suede? Removing or reducing the animal products on your plate inevitably raises questions about what you wear and what other products you have in your life.

There is a world of fun to be had with making vegan choices outside of food.

Choosing to live vegan inspires you to think about provenance and sustainability. It can be hard to navigate at first, but as you discover new products, you'll get to find new favorites that are often better for you and the planet, too. By meeting new vegan friends along the way, you can swap recommendations. For example, who knew that some deodorant isn't vegan? Well, now we do. But as well as having deodorants that haven't been tested on animals, we also get to avoid aluminium, which is in lots of main brand deodorants. And who knew that eau de toilette isn't typically vegan either? Now we have found new favorite scents, which are ethical and come in reusable glass bottles, so they are more sustainable, too. Your new favorite products are just waiting to be found—let us be your guides!

However, you might not be worried about this way of vegan living right now, and prefer to focus only on eating vegan food. We totally support you in that choice! As we have learned, reducing or removing meat and dairy is one of the most effective—if not, the most effective—ways of having a positive impact on the environment, and so by all means leave it at that. But if you are interested, now or in the future, in how to make the most out of this new way of thinking, then read on.

CLOTHES

There's nothing more personal than your choice of clothes. Keep it that way!

When we first cut out animal products, we made zero changes to our wardrobes. Zip. Zilch. Nada. The move to a more plant-based and sustainable diet is an incredibly powerful one, and there is nothing to say that it must be accompanied by a change in your clothing, too. Keep your wardrobe as you wish. And be happy wearing what you want to make you feel great.

Since we're exploring how to reduce animal products in our diet, we'll look at how to avoid animal products in your clothes, too. But please don't think you have to change your wardrobe overnight or throw away the clothes you love. Very few people have the money to do that, and many of us have items of clothing that we've owned and loved for years. Throwing out your old clothes just to buy new ones isn't a very sustainable move! For us, it has been a slower process of replacing clothes as they have worn out with more ethical alternatives.

STREAMLINE YOUR WARDROBE

You don't need to have a minimalist wardrobe in order to wear vegan-friendly clothes. But reducing the number of clothes you have means you can think more deeply about the sustainability and environmental impact of the items you buy and wear. For us, it didn't happen straightaway; but over the course of several years and many house moves, we went through a gradual process of review, remove, replace.

There are plenty of people who will love the clothes that you don't love anymore. Build a box full of clothes that can be worn by someone else. Friends and family may be grateful for your old clothes, as will charity shops. Or find a sustainable fashion shop, where people can exchange "pre-loved" clothing—a much-needed antidote to today's "fast fashion" culture.

Focus instead on having clothes that are well-made and have little negative impact on the world in terms of their environmental footprint and the people who make them. We live in a world of cheap, throwaway fashion. It's far better to have fewer but better-quality items that you really love and that you'll keep for longer.

ANIMAL-FREE CLOTHING

What do we mean by animal-free and cruelty-free clothing? This is clothing—including shoes, wallets, bags, and other accessories, like belts, ties, hats, and bandanas—that has not caused any harm to any animal at any stage of its production process.

If you want to find animal-free clothing, it can be hard to know where to start. Try to shop from brands that are PETA approved (they will display the PETA logo on their website).

{ *PeTA* - A P P R O V E D
VEGAN }

Avoid materials you know to be from animals, and buy clothes that use dyes that have not been tested on animals.

We also support Fair Trade clothing, which means the people who have made the clothes at every stage of their process work under approved conditions and receive fair pay and holidays.

Recently, there has been a huge push toward environmentally positive manufacturing processes, too. This includes using sustainable, natural fabrics and dyes that do not contain harsh chemicals.

It is almost impossible to gather all this information only from reading the label on your clothes! But a bit of research online will produce lots of fashion brands that are supporting these aims. To start off with, here is a list of the main animal-derived materials to avoid.

Fur, leather, and any other animal skin

Most leather is produced as part of the meat and dairy industry, whereas animals are usually raised specifically to be killed for their fur. As well as obviously being bad for the animals, the leather production process is actually very dirty, using lots of harsh chemicals that are harmful to the environment.

We don't wear leather shoes, but we understand that it's up to everyone how they choose to dress. We're not saying get rid of the clothes you have and love! Just be aware of provenance and maybe think more carefully about what you buy in the future.

There are loads of vegan alternatives to both leather and fur. Some vegan leathers are plastic, which are less sustainable, but are widely available. Other eco-friendly leathers are made from things like pineapple or mushroom. Fake fur is easy to find in mainstream retailers. Some people think wearing imitation fur and leather promotes the real thing, but we don't think perfection should get in the way of progress. If purchasing these products diverts money away from the real thing, then that's a step in the right direction!

Wool, angora, and cashmere
These come from sheep, rabbits, and goats, respectively. Although sheep aren't killed for their wool, they grow it for a reason! It helps protect them and keep them warm. Sheep often have their tails clipped off and are tagged or marked as part of the farming process. Rabbits are usually killed for their shearling (the skin with its fur still attached). There are some great synthetic alternatives that will keep you warmer and are quicker and easier to wash and dry. There are also some good natural alternatives, too. We opt for cotton sweaters instead!

Silk
Silk is made by silkworms—a type of caterpillar. They produce long strands of silk in their cocoons, which are boiled (with the pupae still inside) so the strands can be extracted. The actual manufacturing process of silk has a huge negative environmental impact, too. There are lots of natural plant fibers available now such as bamboo—as well as synthetic alternatives—that have the same soft texture but without the cruelty.

Feather/down
We didn't tend to wear many feathers even when we ate meat! But feathers are one of the most common fillings used for cushions, pillows, duvets, and in some super-warm coat linings. The feathers are usually plucked from live birds, as part of the food industry. Many retailers stock vegan versions of them nowadays—just ask.

THE STORY OF IAN'S LEATHER JACKET

We were about six months into our journey as **BOSH!**, and things were going really well. We were releasing videos every day, the Facebook channel was gaining thousands of new followers every week, and we were racking up millions of views. But around that time somebody told me that if we intended to carry on building **BOSH!** as part of the vegan movement, I would have to stop wearing my leather jacket. Initially, this really annoyed me. "Who is this person to tell me what to wear?" I thought. "I've had that jacket for 10 years and it means a lot to me."

Let me tell you a little bit about this jacket. In my twenties I worked in a top-end men's clothing store. At the time, it was one of the best shops in the country. We stocked all the best brands, and fashion-conscious guys from all over the country would come to the store to buy clothes. In my time working in fashion, I amassed a huge collection of great menswear. And one of the items of clothing I acquired was a black leather trucker. It was a sample piece that was given to me by a Levi's sales rep. The jacket never went into production, which meant mine was one of maybe four in the whole world. It was a really simple, high-quality jacket and I loved it. People literally came up to me and asked if they could buy the jacket. It was as cool as they come, was worth a lot of money, and had a very personal backstory so, as I'm sure you can imagine, it pained me to put it in my wardrobe for the last time.

I still have the jacket and I'll probably keep it forever, but I won't ever wear it again because it's not in line with my morals. I still have a couple of old leather belts from my pre-vegan days, although the days I wear them are now few and far between. Good vegan belts can be hard to find! But they're out there if you look for them. I have a couple of old travel bags that have leather straps, but I tend not to use them anymore. I've opted for newer, vegan bags and rucksacks instead.

Since going vegan I've not actually bought anything leather, and I don't plan to. While it feels like leather's everywhere, actually with a bit of research you can find ethical, sustainable versions of almost everything.

JEWELRY

Most jewelry is animal-free, but here are a few things to bear in mind.

Pearls: Most pearls are not naturally found but are "cultured" instead. This means oysters are kept in large farms and irritants inserted into their shells, forcing them to produce pearls. They usually die in the process of having their pearls removed.

Glues: Check with the producer to make sure that they use glues that have not been tested on animals—and that do not contain animal products. This information can be hard to find, sometimes, so do what you can and don't worry if you can't confirm it all!

Fair Trade: The silver and gold industries—as well as the mining for diamonds and other gemstones—are notorious for their poor working conditions and negative environmental impact. There are plenty of Fair Trade–approved suppliers now, so from an ethical standpoint you might want to source your jewelry from one that has been certified.

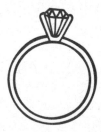

WHERE TO START

The easiest way to get guaranteed animal-free clothes is to hunt down brands that specialize in vegan or cruelty-free clothing. You can easily find out this information online, since most vegan-friendly brands are keen to shout about it! There are some amazing choices available—it's not all about long flowy shirts and dresses these days. Instagram is a great place to look, too. Since some big names in Hollywood have started to follow plant-based eating, the fashion world has followed suit.

Browsing online, chatting in forums, or asking your friends can all help you identify which brands are best for sourcing animal-free clothing. And of course, the best way is to simply walk into a store and ask the assistant to help you find vegan, plant-based clothes.

The other way to know if clothes are free from animals is to read the label and work it out yourself. To do this you need to know which materials are and aren't vegan.

VEGAN-APPROVED FABRICS

Our clothes are basically all cotton. Whether it's cotton, linen, denim, or canvas, basically everything is derived from cotton. T-shirts, shirts, shorts, trousers, jeans, sandals, the lot.

Cotton is fairly water-intensive to produce, so not without its own carbon footprint, but at the end of the day we have to wear something! So it's more important to be respectful of your clothes and make them last. Other than that, we have a few bits that are made from polyester—or a mix of cotton and polyester. Polyester is a plastic, though, so make it last. And consider passing old clothes on when you are done with them, rather than throwing them away.

Previously, alternatives to animal-derived fabrics were all made from plastics, which are not great from a sustainability perspective. But now there are all manner of exciting alternatives available, and many more in development. We're excited whenever we hear about new cruelty-free options. Here are some of our favorites:

- **Organic Fair Trade cotton**—We love this stuff. We like to know that farmers are being looked after and that farming practices are as environmentally friendly as possible. Organic cotton uses fewer chemicals, pesticides, and fertilizers to help the health of the soil. It's also good to see that there are so many recycled brands available now.

- **Linen**—This may make you think of an English gentleman abroad, but it's a very eco-conscious fabric, especially if you source Fair Trade.

- **Hemp and bamboo**—Both are natural fabrics that usually don't involve pesticides or harsh chemicals. Just watch out for rayon, which is made from bamboo but does involve a chemical-intensive production process.

- **Tencel®**—This is super cool! It's also known as lyocell and is made from wood celluose (literally wood pulp!). It has very eco-conscious production processes, as it reuses a lot of the water and chemicals.

- There are also a load of brands making cool things out of fully recycled goods. You can find sneakers, T-shirts, tracksuits, and swimsuits made entirely from recycled plastic bottles! We love getting our hands on bits like that, as they give you an extra spring in your step when you wear them. It's hard to avoid telling people that you are literally wearing old plastic bottles!

Overall, when it comes to clothes, we think people should make their own choices. Add good-quality items to your wardrobe when you feel you need them. Decide how far you want to delve into the world of vegan stuff. It's your call.

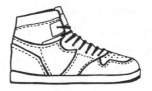

SHOES

So many shoes, both men's and women's, are made with things like suede and leather, so it can be a bit of a struggle to find a vegan version.

Leather and the glues used to make some shoes are both derived from animals. Luckily, there are tons of vegan alternatives available now, made both from synthetic and natural fabrics. Vegan-friendly shoes may display the Vegan Trademark, or a brand may tell you that they are vegan. There are often accidentally vegan shoes you can find, just by asking.

Over time we've found new favorite shoes. Henry likes to wear barefoot shoes (although they hurt his feet a bit!) and Ian likes to wear Converse as he's *that* trendy. EmJ wears sneakers and boots generally (of the cowboy and rocker variety), sandals for lazy days, and high heels for posh do's. All are vegan!

When it comes to your shoes, we recommend starting slowly. Wear the shoes you already have! But when it comes to buying new ones, we recommend replacing them with vegan options. Have a quick google or ask around to find animal-free options. You may just discover new brands that you love. We did!

BUYING SECONDHAND

Shopping in thrift or secondhand stores is the most obvious way for you to develop a truly personal style while keeping costs down and minimizing your impact on the environment.

Buying something secondhand is always a much more sustainable choice, whether it's a vegan-friendly product or not. You're making use of items that already exist rather than producing an entirely new one and throwing the old one away. It means that you're not telling the producer to create more of that item, so it doesn't technically contribute to an increase in demand.

There are some people who say that as the item already exists and it's not part of the usual supply-and-demand chain, it's OK to buy or wear secondhand nonvegan items, like leather. However, wearing any kind of animal product—and some people argue that even wearing fake versions of animal products—helps spread the idea that it is desirable. If someone sees you wearing that secondhand leather jacket and thinks it looks great, it might encourage them to buy a new version for themselves.

There's also the fact that you are wearing something that—even if it was a long time ago—caused harm and suffering to animals . . .

MAKEUP AND SKINCARE

We all worry about what we put into our bodies, but it wasn't until we went vegan that we started to think about what we put *on* our bodies. When we started to look into it, we were surprised to learn just how many animal products can be found in our bathroom cabinets—from moisturizers, soaps, and shower gels to makeup and cosmetics. And, of course, many leading brands are still testing on animals. Even if the item is technically vegan because it doesn't *contain* any animal products, we don't consider it to be truly vegan if its production process has involved cruelty to animals.

But, as more and more people turn toward a more plant-based, animal-free diet, there has been a similar surge in the release of vegan cosmetics in recent years.[110] As a result, there are lots of amazing vegan products available now. From mainstream chains like the Body Shop to higher-end brands, there are products for every price range and many are certified cruelty-free.

Henry's fiancée, EmJ, is one of the UK's leading makeup artists, specializing in vegan makeup for top brands and celebrity clients. Indeed, we're often made up by her for photo shoots and TV—it's not exactly our area of expertise! She's helped educate us, and she's kindly shared her beauty tips with us here.

FIRST OF ALL, WHAT'S THE DIFFERENCE?

First things first, let's get clear about what it means for a product to be vegetarian, vegan, or cruelty-free.

Vegetarian
This product is claiming to not contain animals, but it might include animal by-products, such as beeswax, lanolin, or goat's milk.

Vegan
This product is claiming to not include any animals or animal by-products.

Cruelty-free
A company that says it is cruelty-free claims not to test ingredients or the final product on animals, nor contract with another company that tests on animals.

A really important thing to note from these definitions is that even if a product is labeled as being vegan, it does not necessarily mean it's cruelty-free. Equally, if a product is cruelty-free it does not automatically mean it's vegan. It is also worth bearing in mind that different certificates vary in their level of oversight and, therefore, how much confidence you can have in them. If you're concerned, do some research.

PARENT COMPANIES

There are many companies that are classed as cruelty-free that do not test on animals, but they are owned by large corporations that do. This is a complicated gray area and it really comes down to making up your own mind about whether you're willing to purchase from companies like this.

On the one hand, we have the power of supply and demand. The more we shop from cruelty-free brands, the more money and attention will be given to them by the larger corporations for them to grow. And, in turn, other cruelty-free brands will grow to try to compete with them. But on the other hand, you'll still be supporting and potentially funding those parent companies that do test on animals. And we think it's also important to support smaller independent brands.

But, like everything, this is your decision—make the choices that are right for you.

HOW CAN YOU KNOW IF A BRAND IS CRUELTY-FREE?

It's great when products are transparent about being cruelty-free. Unfortunately there are currently no clear laws on what qualifies a brand to make this claim. A brand can state that they are vegetarian, vegan, or cruelty-free on their website or packaging even if it is not true. Here are three helpful pointers:

STEP 1. DOES THE BRAND SELL IN CHINA?

Current law states that any product that is stocked in China must go through animal testing before it is deemed safe to sell, or it can be pulled off the shelf at random to be tested. This law is due to change in 2020, but at the time of writing, any brand that sells within China cannot currently be classed as "cruelty-free." Many brands will make statements like "We do not test on animals," but be careful with this claim as even though the brands themselves are not testing on animals, they may be using a third party to do it for them. A good way to find out is by going to the brand website and searching for Chinese retailers.

STEP 2. DOES THE BRAND HAVE A CRUELTY-FREE BADGE ON ITS PRODUCTS OR WEBSITE?

Cruelty-free certifications are awarded to brands that have made a pledge to not test on animals. All certifications usually insist that the brand does not test its products or ingredients on animals, or allow a third party to do so.

It is also required to pledge that its suppliers do not test on animals either. Some certifications insist the suppliers give proof that they do not test on animals, some are regularly audited, and some only award certifications to brands that are not owned by a parent company that tests on animals. These requirements are developing over time, so if it is something you would like to know more about, you can find lots of information about individual logos online. A good source is www.ethicalelephant.com. There's a lot to learn!

Below are the most trusted logos you will see in mainstream stores. Note, though, that these logos and the term "cruelty-free" does not mean the product is necessarily vegan or even vegetarian. It concerns the use of animal testing only and could still contain animal products.

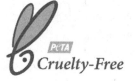

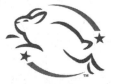

STEP 3. I CAN'T FIND A BADGE—DOES THIS MEAN IT'S NOT CRUELTY-FREE?

Absolutely not! Many brands simply don't yet have the accreditations. Perhaps they can't afford the fees that many organizations charge to use their logo, or they just haven't been awarded the badges yet—it can take a while to be approved. If you love a product or brand, can't find a badge, and can't see if they are selling in China, then there are some trusty cruelty-free search engines to try next:

Websites
- Leaping Bunny: www.leapingbunny.org/guide/brands/list
- Cruelty-free Kitty: www.crueltyfreekitty.com/
- Ethical Elephant: www.ethicalelephant.com
- Logical Harmony: www.logicalharmony.net

Apps
- Bunny Free from PETA
- Cruelty Cutter by Beagle Freedom Project
- Happy Bunny

NOW I KNOW WHICH OF MY PRODUCTS ARE CRUELTY-FREE, WHICH ONES ARE VEGAN-FRIENDLY?

Is there a badge on the packaging or on the website?
It would be wonderful if every vegan product had a reliable badge that we could trust. As time goes on, more and more brands are applying vegan-friendly logos on packaging or on websites, which is brilliant. Here are some to look out for:

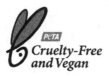

Does the brand's website state it's vegan?

Head to the brand website—is there a vegan section? If not, find the product and head to the description. Most vegan products will state that they are, loud and proud. This is not the most reliable way to ensure it's definitely vegan—it's simply the brand's own claim—but they are under increasing scrutiny, so it's unlikely to be false.

Check the ingredients

We don't do much makeup shopping, but we can tell you that if you are still not 100% sure your product is vegan, as with food items, take a closer read of the labels and work out what the ingredients are.

The main ingredients to watch out for in skincare, makeup and beauty products are honey and animal fats—and some red colorings, which, as in food, are sometimes made from crushed beetles.

We've made a list over the following pages of the key items you're likely to find in your toiletries and makeup, and what to look out for in them. We've also included a handy list of ingredients on page 268 to check your products against.

SKINCARE

Cleansers, face washes, and scrubs

Beeswax, also known as "cera alba," is often found in face washes, as is lanolin, which is derived from sheep sweat. You are likely to see stearic acid, too. This is a bit of a trickier one, as stearic acid *can* now be found in a vegan-friendly form, however it's originally made from animal fats, so if in doubt check it out online.

Serums and moisturizers

You may have heard of hyaluronic acid. It's a magic ingredient that is suppposed to minimize pores and speed up cell renewal. But beware, as some hyaluronic acid is derived from cockerel combs or other animal tissues. Luckily, though, there is a vegan version now available and a lot of products use this instead.

Other common ingredients found in serums and moisturizers are tallow, which is rendered animal fat, animal collagen, animal glycerin, and animal squalene, extracted from the livers of sharks. This is not to be confused with squalane, which is from olives! Retinol (another common ingredient) can be found in both animal and vegan forms, so do check to make sure.

Shower gels, soaps, and body scrubs

Honey and lanolin can often be found in body washes to soften the skin. Stearic acid is often used in soaps, in both animal and plant forms, so do check. Many scrubs used to contain plastic microbeads, which found their way into our water system. However, thanks to campaigners, these are now illegal in the UK and US.

HAIRCARE

Hairstyling products

Beeswax is a common ingredient due to its strength. Another common one is glycerin, although this can also come in a plant-based form. Stearic acid, which can come from animal fats, is another one to avoid.

Shampoo and conditioner

Many shampoos and conditioners contain lanolin and honey to give softness. Other common ingredients include keratin to help strengthen and smooth hair, which is derived from ground-up animal hooves and horns. Guanine, from fish scales, can be included to give shine. Also look out for stearic acid, although this can also come in plant form.

MAKEUP

Foundation and concealers

These provide the perfect base for your makeup, and many claim to be silky smooth. So you may find real silk in your foundation! This is made using silkworms by the thousands. You also may find lanolin, beeswax, animal-based glycerin, or honey.

Mascara

There are lots of vegan mascaras on the market now. However, a fair amount still contain animal-based glycerin and guanine, which is derived from fish scales. Beeswax and honey are common, too.

Eye shadows and eye pencils

Many brands are turning to vegan formulations, but the biggest animal-based ingredient sneaking into eye shadow and pencils is the cochineal beetle, also known as "carmine." Beeswax is also commonly found in pencils and cream eye shadow.

Face powders (blushers, bronzers, and highlighters)

Silk and pearls are often used in powders to help with blending. Carmine from the cochineal beetle is often found in powders with a lot of color. You may even find some of our fishy friends—guanine—used to create a shimmery effect.

Lipstick, gloss, and balm

There are endless kinds of lip products available, but sadly it's also the product type most likely not to be vegan-friendly. Many lip products have red pigments in them, so cochineal is a common ingredient. Beeswax and guanine are also common ingredients. Synthetic and plant-based colorings are available though.

Nail polishes and gels

Most nail polishes contain animal products, either to add color or shimmer or to hydrate or strengthen your nails. The shimmer is often from guanine. Shellac is derived from the secretion of female lac bugs in India and is used in most gel polishes and occasionally in regular polish. You are also likely to find carmine for color and keratin, which is made from animal horns and hooves, for nail strengthening.

OTHER ITEMS

Deodorants

Henry in particular has taken on the challenge of testing out every vegan and natural deodorant he ever finds. The winners are usually salt-based. In nonvegan deodorants you will often find beeswax and glycerin—although glycerin can also be plant-derived. The main issue is that most deodorant brands are owned by big companies that also sell in China, so, until the law changes (see page 259), will have been tested on animals.

Toothpaste

As with deodorants, the main issue with most brands is that they are stocked in China so, sadly, are likely to be tested on animals. And a lot of toothpastes contain glycerin. Glycerin comes in both animal and plant form so the only way of knowing is by asking the brand or looking out for that sticker.

CHEAT SHEET

Nonvegan ingredients to watch out for [111]

adrenaline*
allantoin*
alpha-hydroxy acids*
ambergris
arachidonic acid
beeswax (cera alba)
biotin*
bone phosphate (E542)
calcium caseinate
calcium lactate*
calcium stearate*
caprylic acid
carmine (carminic acid)
castor
castoreum
cerebrosides
cetyl alcohol
chitosan
cholesterol
civet
cochineal
collagen*
cystine*

disodium inosinate*
emu oil
gelatin
glycerin*
guanine
honey
hyaluronic acid*
keratin
L-cysteine*
lactitol
lactose
lanolin
lard
lecithin
linoleic acid
magnesium stearate*
mink oil
monoglycerides, glycerides*
musk*
myristic acid*
oestrogen (estradiol or
    estrogen)*
oleic acids*

palmitic acid*

panthenol (provitamin B5 and derivatives)*

polypeptides*

polysorbates*

pristane*

progesterone*

propolis

retinol*

RNA*

royal jelly

shellac (E904)

silk powder

snails

squalene (not squalane, which comes from plants)

stearic acid*

turtle oil

urea (uric acid)

vitamin A (retinol)*

vitamin D3 (cholecalciferol)*

* Indicates that a plant-based alternative with the same name is available for this ingredient. Frustratingly, labels don't usually say whether an ingredient is plant-based or not, so the only way to be sure is to check the website or ask the brand directly.

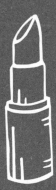

A NOTE ON BRUSHES

Makeup and shaving brushes are often made from animal hair—including mink, squirrel, goat, and badger to name a few—as they are traditionally thought to buff makeup more effectively. Many brush brands say that the brushes are made from "natural hair," which, in other words, means animal hair.

Besides the hair itself, you could also find nonvegan friendly glue holding the brushes together. Opt for synthetic alternatives instead. Brushes using synthetic fabrics also hold fewer bacteria and less dirt than animal hair.

False lashes
This is often an overlooked one, but many lash brands use animal as well as human hair—choose "synthetic" or "faux mink" or "faux silk" and, even better, go with an accredited vegan and cruelty-free brand.

Sanitary products
Most sanitary towels and tampons are not cruelty-free. They may contain chlorine or other chemicals tested on animals. In addition, pads and plastic applicators are usually single-use. Reusable menstrual cups and applicators are available, though, and more eco-friendly period products are coming onto the market, so look out for those.

Hair removal

One item we were most surprised about was our razors! Sometimes the moisturizing gel strips contain animal products—and many manufacturers test other products on animals, even if they don't actually test the razors on animals, so this is quite a complex one! Luckily, there are many vegan-friendly razors, shaving creams, and after balms now.

Waxing is not generally vegan-friendly as the wax can contain chemicals or perfumes and some contain beeswax—although most are plant-based or made from paraffin. Some also contain honey and other animal products. Sugaring is generally considered the vegan's hair removal method of choice! But there are vegan alternatives to waxes available if you seek them out. We'd also like to stress though that hair removal is a completely personal choice and we are in no way saying this should be an essential part of your routine!

Perfume and aftershaves

Traditionally, many perfumes and aftershaves include civet or musk. These ingredients are derived from the secretions of civet cats and musk deer. These don't actually even need to be included on the labels, as the ingredients are often described as "secret formulas." Thankfully, these ingredients are much less common now and synthetic versions are being used instead. Other nonvegan ingredients to watch out for are leather, honey, and beeswax, which are all used mainly for their scent. Look out for the trusted Vegan badge (see page 262).

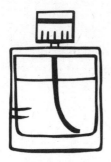

Sunscreen

This can often contain many of the same animal-based ingredients as cleansers: beeswax, lanolin, collagen, and stearic acid, so always check the label. Also look out for elastin and chitin, which is often made from crustacean shells.

Dopp kits and makeup bags

These are usually either expensive and made from leather, or cheap and made from plastic. When we turned vegan it was things like this that needed a little more thought. There are some great alternatives available made of Piñatex and cork, usually handmade by independent designers, and EmJ makes her own at www.emjcompany.com.

Treatments

Treatments (things like facials, massages, or manicures) are typically not vegan. As we learned on page 267, nail polishes are generally not vegan. Many facial products and massage oils will contain nonvegan products, too. If that's something that you want to think about, then by all means ask before you go for the treatment. There are places that do cater to vegan treatments, either because all their products are already vegan, or they can make changes at your request.

TATTOOS

The ink used in tattoos can often contain bone char, animal fats, glycerin, or shellac, but it's totally possible to use vegan-friendly inks, so just ask. The other thing to be aware of is that the papers used for the stencils can contain lanolin, and some of the aftercare products may contain animal products, too.

So if you're thinking of inking up, we recommend you head to a vegan-friendly tattoo studio so there's one less thing to worry about . . .

As always, the internet is your friend, so research and ask for recommendations.

As far as we are concerned, we don't worry about this too much. The key thing is to make living vegan easy for yourself, especially when you are getting started. It's better to take small steps rather than to immediately try to make sure every single thing is vegan. But if in doubt, ask.

RANDOM THINGS THAT CONTAIN ANIMAL PRODUCTS

Money
Some banknotes around the world—including in the UK, Australia, and Canada—contain tallow, an animal fat that is used to give the bills their smooth texture.

Condoms
Many latex condoms use casein (milk protein) in the manufacturing process to make them more comfortable. The ingredients have also often been tested on animals, and use some harsh chemicals in their production. Luckily, there are plenty of vegan-friendly condoms available now, including from the big brands. Phew! Look for the Vegan Society badge.

Craft supplies
Paints and paintbrushes, glues, crayons, and even paper can all contain products derived from animals. Most acrylic paints tend to be vegan-friendly, but do check online to make sure—there are some great vegan craft websites that list all the major brands and detail which are vegan and which aren't.

Chlorine

A bit like the plastic issue we discuss on page 286, chlorine is an example of how it's almost impossible to live completely, 100% vegan. Chlorine is tested on animals, so you may wish to avoid this where you can. The main culprits are swimming pools, cleaning products, and tampons, but we're not saying you can't have a dip on your summer vacation or should give up your favorite exercise. Choose organic or vegan-approved tampons, as these will be chlorine-free. And see page 278 for more on cleaning products.

Vitamins

Some vitamin pills are coated with gelatin, which is an animal product, so look for vitamins that are vegan-friendly. Obviously, avoid fish oils. Some children's vitamins can be colored, so make sure they use vegan-friendly dyes. Most of the big brands have products made with vegans in mind so it's easy to find good alternatives.

Candles

Beeswax candles are an obvious no, but beware that most candles contain some kind of animal fat to help them harden. And some even contain oils from whales and dolphins. Cheap paraffin wax candles are not a good alternative though, as they contain high levels of toxic chemicals. Some candles are made from palm oil, which is not a very animal-friendly ingredient (see page 161), so try organic soy—which also burns for much longer, too.

THE VEGAN HOME

Once you've reviewed your wardrobe and bathroom, you can start looking at other parts of your home life.

Be aware that your home is almost guaranteed to be filled with products that aren't vegan. Think back to the Vegan Society's definition of "as far as is possible and practicable" and that applies more than ever here. You simply cannot be 100% vegan in your home—not easily anyway. Even books will typically be bound with glue that is not vegan. Parts of your furniture may not be vegan, and the way the technology in your home was manufactured may also not be strictly vegan. Your mattress may contain wool—many do—although there are now some vegan mattresses available to buy.

When we started on our journey, we hadn't even thought about how the things in our homes could potentially use animal products. This is where you need to exercise your personal choice and make some decisions, or just accept that you are happy as you are.

Don't beat yourself up if there are things that are not vegan in your house.

The things that you keep forever—or for a long time anyway—and aren't replaced on a regular basis will have less of an impact than those things which you buy regularly. We would much rather you stick with a vegan (or more of a vegan) diet and be happy with all your existing things, than get obsessed with only having vegan products in your house and then give up because it's all too hard.

With that in mind though, let's take a look at some of the most common household items:

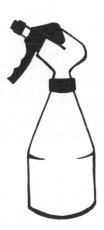

HOUSEHOLD CLEANING PRODUCTS

There are lots of natural cleaning products available now, so you can easily avoid using those containing harsh chemicals such as bleach and chlorine. This doesn't automatically mean they are cruelty-free though. We use a vegan dishwashing liquid now because someone once saw a nonvegan brand on our Instagram story and called us out on it. We're always learning, too! Many cleaning products also contain beeswax or lanolin, so check the ingredients. Real feather dusters are an obvious no-no! And we also try to avoid using disposable sponges, instead using ones that can be washed and reused.

BEDDING

Where you can, choose organic, vegan-friendly duvets, pillows, and throws. Organic cotton uses far fewer chemicals than traditionally processed cotton, so its environmental footprint is much smaller. There are some amazing eco-friendly bedding suppliers now that use low-impact production processes and dyes, and use natural and biodegradable materials, including bamboo, coconut husk, and linen.

It goes without saying, really, that you should avoid feather or down-stuffed pillows and duvets, silk sheets, and wool blankets (see page 247 for more on these fabrics).

RUGS AND SOFAS

It's not just that the leather in sofas is nonvegan, it is also likely to be heavily treated with resins and preservatives, so its negative impact on the environment is much higher than vegan alternatives. Opt for leather-, wool-, and silk-free options when shopping for homeware. Lots of big retailers stock vegan collections now. There are some great alternative vegan fabrics available, including faux fur and faux leather, but beware that some are less sustainable than others. Acrylic is a plastic, so try to use natural fabrics where you can, such as cotton or linen. You can even get rugs made from recycled bottles![112]

PRINTING

Books, magazines, and home printing: it's the ink that is the main concern here, as many contain animal products including glycerin, bone char, and shellac. There are some vegan-approved alternatives available, made from vegetable-based dyes, but they're not all that easy to come by, and we have found that they aren't compatible with most home printers. We advise you to print only when necessary and also look into printer cartridges that can be refilled, rather than replaced and thrown away.

Make sure the paper is sustainably sourced and/or recycled. Look for the FSC logo, which ensures the product you are buying will help keep forests alive for future generations, as well as supporting the rights of indigenous populations.

ELECTRONIC GOODS

We love our laptops and smartphones as much as the next millennial, but we were quite shocked to learn how many animal products are used in their production. LCD screens may contain animal products, and gelatin is used as part of the manufacture of some batteries. Then there are the plastics and glues used in the electronic boards inside.

One other issue to think about when it comes to almost all electronic goods is that the mining of the necessary rare-earth elements tends to be damaging to the environment and exploitative of the workers involved. As with everything, it's almost impossible in the Western world we live in to totally avoid any social or environmental impact from our electronics, but we think it's good to be aware of these issues so you can make an informed decision about whether you really do need that next upgrade or not . . .

ENERGY SUPPLIERS

Green and renewable energy is obviously a great step in the right direction, but just because it is renewable, doesn't mean it's necessarily vegan. One of the most exciting new developments in green energy is anaerobic digestion, where microorganisms digest waste material and produce biogas. This also goes a long way to reducing our landfill. However, it's not vegan. Ecotricity is the UK's first certified vegan energy provider, and hopefully more will follow suit soon. [113]

PETS

Whether or not vegans should keep animal companions is a hot topic. Some say that since pets are purely for their owners" enjoyment, keeping a pet is not in keeping with vegan ideals. Others say that if you are rescuing the animal, then it's helping out an animal in need and so is perfectly OK—it is, in fact, a positive act.

There is even some sensitivity around the terminology of "keeping" pets—some people believe no human should "own" another animal, and so some vegans who have animals in their homes consider them to be an equal part of their family as any other member. Some choose to call them "animal friends" to reflect this position.

There's also the issue of breeding. Many animals, and in particular dogs, have been intensively bred over the years to develop specific attributes that are appealing to humans. Many of the dogs that have become fashionable recently— including flat-faced dogs like pugs and bulldogs, small dogs like dachshunds and other, larger breeds like Dalmatians— suffer from health issues as a result of their breeding. These most often include breathing problems, blindness, and deafness, as well as hip and other joint issues, which can have a serious impact on their day-to-day life. Purebred cats also suffer from similar genetic defects. Many ways in which animals are bred are also considered to be ethically dubious, including "puppy mills" and other mass-produced breeding programs.

For this reason, a common position is "adopt, don't shop," since adopting helps rescue animals who are in need of help, and moves business away from breeders. Only you can decide where you stand on this.

When it comes to feeding your pets, you can get good vegan-approved pet foods for almost all common domestic animals. Beware that some animals, however, such as snakes and cats, can only eat animal products.

We love animals, but we don't have pets. Ian loves cats—and fully identifies as a "cat person"—but he won't get one because they're obligate carnivores and he doesn't want to feed one meat! When he was younger Henry had cats and loved them, but he was super allergic unfortunately, and still is. We LOVE dogs, and every now and again our housemate Anna will bring over the most delightful dog called Barney. We have long, regular discussions about getting a **BOSH!** doggie. It's definitely something we want to do, but we are just waiting for the right time.

An interesting question is whether owning animals as a child encourages a wider love for all animals in later life. Maybe. Animals are loads of fun, but a big resonsibility! But if you had a childhood dog that you loved like a member of your family, then you may realize that a baby pig is very much like a baby doggie. Yet for some reason (maybe tradition?) we choose to eat one but love the other!

Overall, we think it's a great thing to rescue animals to give them a new home, as long as you treat that animal with the respect they deserve.

CARS AND TRANSPORT

Unfortunately most cars aren't vegan. It's a good example of how being vegan is a direction to move in rather than an absolute. Avoiding leather seats is the number one step when looking for a vegan car. Be aware that there will be some animal parts used in any liquid crystal displays, and the steel for the car's frame may have been lubricated with animal fat. At this stage, there's not a lot you can do about that, but by all means let manufacturers know you are looking for animal-product-free cars, and the more requests they get, the more likely they are to listen! In addition to the seats and the interior detail, you can select vegan tires. Some tires contain animal products, but mainstream brands are starting to stock vegan tires, so definitely ask.

Another big thing to think about with a car, is the question of gasoline. Obviously we know that gas is not good for the environment and creates emissions. It's also worth considering how the gas was sourced, which will no doubt have involved drilling and loss of animal life.

Ultimately, we believe everyone is going to drive electric cars in the relatively near future. Yes, they are still using power, and yes, there is still work to do on the batteries, but we believe the quicker we can all move to electric cars, the better. So if you can, do.

Or even better, avoid driving a car altogether. We try to cycle around London whenever we can, and will happily trade a 30-minute drive for a bike ride instead. Nipping around on cycles is such a freeing way to travel: it's fun and has the added fitness bonus! And, of course, if you are lucky enough to live in a place with decent public transport, then use it. You'll be doing your bit for the environment and probably saving money.

The big one, though, is flying. We've already covered the impact of flying in this book (see page 36). We're not going to tell you to flat-out not use airplanes. Have you tried traveling between the UK and North America by boat? It's not really practical. Be aware that the cost to the environment is huge, and obviously the manufacture of a plane is not a vegan process, not to mention the damage caused to animals by planes and airports. Just think sensibly about flying, and where possible, go for more environmentally sustainable and planet-friendly options. Trains and boats can be fun.

That said, all of this is your call. We're not going to tell you how to live your life. Travel is important, and exploring different cultures, communities, and ways of life helps expand our minds and bring us together. It helps us develop as human beings. Travel as you need, but try to be as sustainable as you can.

PLASTIC

There is no escaping that plastic is a huge issue right now. Single-use plastics are known to be one of the biggest threats to our marine environment. In the UK, 2.5 billion coffee cups (coated with a thin film of polyethylene) are thrown away each year,[114] and only 0.25% are recycled.[115] Then there are the plastic water bottles, the plastic used in the packaging for all our household products, food items, and medicines, plastic wrap, plastic bags, the plastic used in our electronics . . . It's endless.

Although most plastics don't contain animal products, some do, and the manufacturing process can also be harmful to animal habitats. The main issue, we think, though is that after you've used your plastic item it generally gets thrown away and what happens next is harder to track. We've all seen the images of marine life getting caught up in plastic waste and heard of sea creatures found with plastic items in their stomachs. Although for anyone interested in the issue of plastic in the ocean, while we don't disagree we should move away from single-use plastic, it is a bit of a distraction. About half of all plastic in the ocean is from fishing nets,[116] and most of the great Pacific Garbage Patch is fishing gear.[117]

Plastic, though, is a really good example of how hard it is to be 100% vegan. We don't think you can ever, truly live a

pure vegan lifestyle because almost everything has either
a direct or indirect impact on animals—fossil fuels are the
by-product of animals, field animals often get harmed in the
harvesting of vegetables, insect repellent can cause distress
to mosquitos . . .

We're not saying all this to stress you out! What we're saying
is that being vegan and living a vegan life is about doing what
you can to live in a way that supports all living creatures.
We use recycled plastic when we can and eco bottles for our
water. Ian even walks around with his own cutlery hanging
off his rucksack (although I'm not sure it's ever been used!).
We love shops where you can take your own containers
and fill them up with food and other items—we're halfway
through a move away from plastic shampoo and conditioner
bottles. And it's great that some supermarkets are starting to
embrace this way of shopping, too.

Thanks to the amount of cooking we do at **BOSH!**, we
order our food online and have it delivered to save time.
Because of this, we end up with more plastic waste than
we'd like. It's far from ideal and we're honest about this.
Our business exists to help people eat vegan. We're
encouraging a lot of people to cut down the amount of
meat they're eating, which in turn is helping them to reduce
their carbon footprint. We're not perfect, but as far as we
can, we try to make choices that will have the most positive
impact on the world we live in.

TRAVEL AND VACATIONS

If you think back to your childhood and your most important memories, we bet a lot revolve around vacations you took with your family. Vacations have provided us both with some of our most treasured memories and most important life lessons.

Traveling, if you can afford it, is a gift. It allows you to experience wonderful moments, open your eyes to different cultures, and become a more well-rounded individual. Just like exploring veganism, you meet new people and see a whole new way of life. Many of our most important moments happened on vacation, so we are firm believers in the power of getting away. And some of the most interesting and forward-thinking people we know are this way because they're well traveled. Vacationing as a vegan though can be challenging, so it's definitely worth a bit of preplanning.

If you are traveling overseas, do some research first. You'll be well catered to in most cities worldwide, so check HappyCow.net, or Vanilla-Bean.com to plan where you'll eat. There are many vegetarian and vegan hotels and B&Bs, too. If you are planning to visit a more remote region, be prepared to take your own snacks, and you might be wise to consider renting a house or cottage so you can cook. Download the Vegan Passport app, which will help you communicate your dietary requirements in 78 languages or buy a paper copy from the Vegan Society. Have a look at the different cuisines we discuss on page 212, too, as there are some areas of the world that are already more on board with the vegan diet.

Henry loves Japan. The first time he went he was a meat eater; the second time he was vegan. And the two trips were wildly different. Traveling around Japan as a vegan was a real learning experience. Even their veggie noodle soups are typically made with fish sauce. Japanese people love eggs so much they will sometimes have a raw egg for breakfast. And they love their raw fish and BBQ food. Finding vegan food in a country where you don't speak the language, can be a challenge.

With a bit of planning and determination, it's possible to make it work. You could even discover a new cuisine like *shojin ryori*, Japan's naturally vegetarian "temple food." Before you go, learn a few basics of the language, enough to explain "no meat, no fish, no dairy, no eggs." Look up vegan restaurants before you go, and have some fun using Google Translate to decode ingredients on supermarket snacks! Remember to order the vegan option on your flight, and pack extra snacks for trips.

It's not just the food to consider though. If you're heading somewhere exotic you may need a vaccine. You should be aware that most vaccines are not vegan! We would always err on the side of caution and advise that you take your doctors" advice. Vaccines save lives—both yours and other people's.

If you're concerned about the carbon footprint of your travels, consider whether you can offset it. There are companies who, for a fee, will plant trees for you, and that will enable you to offset your flight's carbon footprint. But be aware that not all of these companies are created equal. Some of them don't ensure the trees grow—they throw seeds out of the window of a helicopter. If you are going to try something like this, then find a company that you are sure will raise the tree properly and ensure it lives to maturity. While many people are offsetting their carbon in this way, not everyone agrees with the principle. The counterargument is that you are simply paying for your indulgences, and that we should be making the effort to live more sustainably in the first place. You have to make the decision that feels right for you.

Here are our top tips for vegan travels:

- **Bring a packed lunch.** We tend to bring our own vegan meals, as typically the vegan options on planes, trains, and boats are rubbish, or nonexistent. Feed yourself, whether you've cooked the food or stopped by a vegan-friendly shop on the way. You'll usually have the added bonus of enjoying a better meal, too!

- **Pack your own vegan cosmetics** (including sunscreen and insect repellent) and take them with you, as you can't guarantee they'll be available where you're going.

- **Get the Vegan Passport app**, which will help you to communicate your food preferences.

- **Read our tips on chatting with waiters** on page 236. Try learning a few basic phrases in the local language, particularly about ordering vegan food, so you are ready to ask for what you want.

- **Make a list of vegan- and veggie-friendly restaurants** in the areas you are going to. You can then share good eating tips with other veggies and vegans on the way or when you get back home.

- Think about the sustainability of your travel options, and if you can, **fly only when necessary**.

- **Speak to your hotel** or place you're staying and let them know you are vegan. Hopefully, they will be able to accommodate you. If not, it's a good reason to try out the nearest vegan lodge or spa (they do exist!).

WHAT NEXT?

You'll get lots of questions. People will wonder why you're eating a different meal at restaurants. When you go round to your friends' houses for dinner they'll ask why you're eating vegan.

You'll talk to your friends and family about what you are doing. You'll find out their opinions and navigate those discussions as tactfully and respectfully as you can. You can be sure that you'll hear their opinions, and you'll get used to the best way to deliver yours!

Do your best to be extra polite and respectful, so you can get your message across without damaging your relationships. Some people are very set in their view of the world, and may take any alternative views as a threat. Navigate that carefully.

You'll learn brief and powerful answers to the most common questions. Before long you'll be able to answer them with ease and conviction. And you'll keep learning.

Paying closer attention to the food that you eat might mean you start to focus on other aspects of your health and well-being, too. Take care of your body. Learn about nutrition and help those around you with tips that you pick up along the way. Cook for your friends and show them how delicious vegan food can be. Become a source of information about where is good to get vegan food near you.

Become a source of inspiration, proud of the decision you've made. Build a new, positive life for yourself and you'll have a powerful effect on those around you.

Steve Paton is a friend of ours who works at the Truman Brewery in East London. He ran food festivals—and the odd rave! In 2015 he made the decision to cut out animal products after watching the documentary *Cowspiracy*. He was absolutely shocked by what he learned in that film. He had no idea that animal products were the leading cause of climate change. And once he discovered that, he couldn't go back.

Steve had a burning passion to do something positive for the world, to do his bit to help reduce climate change and animal suffering. He saw how inherently positive the vegan movement was, and also noticed how it was starting to unite people from different cultures and backgrounds in London. He wanted to support this movement, and also help to promote and unite the people who were involved.

Along with Rudi Khalastchi, Jordon Taylor, their team, and the support of the Truman Brewery, Steve developed Vegan Nights into what it is today: London's biggest and best plant-based food festival and party.

The first event had space for about 500 people. Over 2,000 turned up. They had queues for half a mile down the road. The team realized they were onto something powerful.

Since September 2017, the event has grown and grown to become the biggest vegan food event in Europe and hosts 4,000 people eight times a year. It brings together people from different ethnicities, sexualities, political preferences, and genders. It's a powerful, multicultural event, that celebrates vegan food in a collaborative, welcoming, nonjudgmental way. Despite its name, it's not only vegans who go. It's a mixture of people from all walks of life, with different eating habits, who want to party together and try vegan.

And what a party. They have dozens of street food vendors serving wonderful and varied vegan dishes. Music plays all night, with DJs, live acts, and performances. We love Vegan Nights so much we launched our cookbook **BISH BASH BOSH!** with them: we performed a live cooking demo and DJ set for thousands of people.

So many people find they embark on a journey of vegan food and then have a burning desire to share what they've learned with the world.

You might find you want to cook food for people. Or you may find you want to build a business that is focused around changing the world in this way. An incredible 87% of people would be willing to buy a product based on the company being an advocate for causes that they believe in.[118] People want to buy from businesses with values that align with their own, so by creating a vegan business you are entering into business with a huge head start.

Another friend of ours, Ellie, found the lack of vegan cheeses to be very, very difficult, so she started to experiment with making her own. As a home cook anyway (she was a nanny in her day job), she became proficient at making delicious vegan cheese. Many of her friends had been put off veganism by exactly the same problem—their love of cheese. With Ellie's incredible recipes they discovered they could get a cheese that satisfied their taste buds. Ellie featured one of her recipes on our recipe channel, and the incredibly gooey CamemBOSH! recipe has since had millions of views. Fast-forward to today, and she's turned this passion into a business and now sells vegan cheese via her Kinda Co.

website. She was a personal inspiration to those around her. And by reducing animal products in your life, you can be, too.

Closer to home, EmJ is a makeup artist who was frustrated that the only makeup bags she could find were leather. She needed them for her work, but didn't want to support the use of animal-based fabrics. She and her mum created a range of makeup bags in her parents' home factory. Today, EmJ Company (www.theemjcompany.com) sells makeup bags, accessories, and more. Top makeup artists carry her kit, and her products are found backstage across the UK.

We're not saying everyone should start up a vegan cheese business or make their own bags, but we want to show you that there's never been a better time to pursue your passion and do something powerful and purposeful with your life. Do what you can to pursue your dream and build something that is geared toward making a better planet, reducing climate change, and helping end animal suffering.

The planet is warming up at a terrifying rate and looks likely to cause further sea level rise, conflict, and catastrophic damage to our environment and the habitats of animals and the world's population. The number one thing we can all do to help slow down or even reverse this damage is to change what we put on our plates. The move toward a more vegan diet—even if it's just a few meals a week—will not only change your impact on the environment, but will also be a positive and powerful move toward showing compassion for all beings on the planet.

By making this change, you start to impact not only yourself, but those around you. You start a ripple effect on the people you come into contact with. By being a positive inspiration, more and more people will start to follow suit. If you support a vegan business, via the process of supply and demand, more and more products will become available that are vegan, meaning more people can eat vegan food. It will become easier and more commonplace. And together we can shift our country, our continent, and ultimately our planet to a healthier, more sustainable, more ethical way of living. But first, start with yourself.

Veganism is not about a pure ideal. The goal is to avoid harming animals, but in modern life it's practically impossible to do that completely; even running, driving cars, or farming vegetables can cause harm to wildlife. That's why the Vegan Society defines veganism as "a way of living that seeks to exclude, as far as is possible and practicable, all forms of exploitation of, and cruelty to animals." This is easier than we might otherwise have thought and leaves room for interpretation—for you to do it your way.

The planet needs you to find your way.

66

Best time to plant a tree? Twenty years ago. Second best time? Today.

ANCIENT CHINESE PROVERB

A FINAL WORD FROM HENRY

In the four years since becoming vegan, my life has completely transformed. At 35, I'm fitter than I've ever been in my life. I'm happier because I've turned my passion into my job. Most important, I wake up every day knowing that I'm pursuing my purpose. Promoting plant-based food has made me into a better, more complete, more empowered person. The funny thing is, I've seen this in nearly everyone I've met who has chosen to be vegan. They become better versions of themselves, more in line with their morals.

Changing our food is the single biggest thing we can do, as individuals, to stop destroying our planet, and if we all start to move in this direction we'll see big changes start to happen really soon. Be the change you wish to see in the world. Fight for what you love. Try eating vegan. And you might just find it's the best decision you ever made in your life, for your health, the planet, and for us all.

"This is the real secret of life—to be completely engaged with what you are doing in the here and now. And instead of calling it work, realize it is play."—Alan Watts, *The Essence of Alan Watts*

A FINAL WORD FROM IAN

Becoming vegan is the best thing that I have ever done. It's the single most important decision I've ever made and will ever make. I've always been a passionate, interested, and loyal person but veganism allowed me to focus my passion, fuel my interests, and enhance my loyalty more than I ever thought possible. It's opened my mind to a way of living that I never thought was possible. It's led me to become more altruistic, loving, and charitable, which in turn has led me to become a fundamentally better person.

Three times a day, at breakfast, lunch, and dinner, I put my beliefs and my values into practice and that's a wonderful thing. Veganism has given me a purpose and, in turn, has given my life meaning that it didn't have before.

I'm going to use the rest of my life to promote veganism to the best of my ability because I wholeheartedly believe it's the most effective weapon in the arsenal we have to fight the war on climate change.

FAQS

Equipping yourself with some well-thought-out answers to some of the most common questions you might get asked means you will feel better prepared for when people want to engage in a conversation about your veganism. Here are the questions we find ourselves being asked most often and the answers we usually provide:

How do you feel about buying from nonvegan companies?

Although it's obviously great that lots of well-known brands and companies are producing vegan products alongside their nonvegan collections, it can be difficult for vegans to reconcile. On the one hand, your money is still going to a company that supports the use of animal products. But on the other, by buying vegan items, even from traditionally nonvegan suppliers, it is increasing the demand for those items, which helps normalize vegan choices and will in turn encourage other companies to advocate for vegan-friendly practices.

I have canine teeth and I'm able to digest meat, so doesn't that mean I am a carnivore?

Our distant ancestors certainly ate meat, but not in the quantities we do today and with not a fraction of the environmental impact our farming methods have on the planet. They also didn't have as much choice. Today, it's perfectly possible to eat a well-balanced, nutritious diet without the need to harm or hurt animals. It's a choice now, rather than a necessity.

What about my children?

This is a huge issue and a source of worry for many parents. The Vegan Society has wonderful resources on enjoying a healthy vegan pregnancy and raising vegan children. There's a question that often gets asked of vegan parents—whether it's OK to force your opinions on your children, perhaps before they can make informed decisions of their own. We completely understand this perspective, and if that's how you feel, then fine! But just as with adults, it's perfectly safe for babies and children to eat a vegan diet—and also for pregnant women. In all instances, the same guidelines apply to making sure they get enough vitamin B12, iron, calcium, and iodine. If this is something you want to pursue, then opt for fortified organic milks and breakfast cereals, plenty of nuts and seeds, whole grains, and green leafy veg. Speak to your doctor to be sure, and they may recommend a daily vitamin pill or drops. Some baby formulas are dairy-based, so make sure to opt for a vegan alternative.

You can't be 100% vegan so what's the point?

It's true. You can never be 100% vegan. First there is the fact that you're bound to slip up at some point, whether that's over traces of milk powder in your potato chips, the glue holding your notebook together, or the wrong pint of lager.

Second, there's the bigger issue that so many manufacturing processes probably somehow, somewhere, have an impact on animals in some way. Whether it's the gas you're using to cook with, the car seat you're sitting on or the pool you swim in at your local community recreation center. Then there's the more involved argument, which is that the soil used to grow our plant-based diets inevitably contains nutrients derived from decayed plants and animal remains. We say, don't beat yourself up about it. Even though you can never be 100% vegan, the decisions you make at mealtimes and how you spend money can ensure that you have a positive impact on your own health, the health of the planet, and on the lives of animals.

Why don't you eat dairy? Surely being vegetarian is enough?

Many people believe that milk and cheese belong in a different category, as does honey, as they don't involve actually consuming the animal. But these food types do still cause animal suffering and are still poor choices from a sustainability perspective. The least sustainable plant-based food choice is still significantly more sustainable than the most sustainable animal-based food choice.[119] So for us, cutting out animal products includes eggs, dairy, and honey.

Isn't moderation OK? What if my mum's made a nonvegan tea? Isn't it better not to waste it?

Moderation is a great way to live your life and we agree that life is all about balance. But some things are clear-cut, and for us, the damage that animal agriculture is doing to the planet is completely unacceptable, so we will never drink a nonvegan tea. But we understand that for many people moderation is a better choice, and if they are in the process of cutting down their meat and dairy intake, then we salute that, however they choose to do it. And we'll keep providing recipes for you all!

You need meat for protein—there just isn't enough protein in plants for the kind of exercise I do. We hear this one *all* the time. But getting enough protein in your diet is really easy. There are many, many delicious, easy-to-find sources of plant-based protein out there. We've listed some of the best sources on page 140. If you're still not convinced, look at Patrik Baboumian, the world-record-holding strongman from Germany. Also known as Popeye, he is 100% vegan! If you really want to keep a close eye on this, use one of the many online trackers to log what you eat.

You can't really thrive without eating meat as you're always going to be deficient in various things.
This is a common misconception. Meat gives you a powerful hit of nutrients and vitamins, it's true, and is also a complete source of protein. But all of these nutrients and vitamins can also be found in plants, apart from two: vitamin D (which we can get from the sun) and B12 (which we get from fortified vegan milks).

It is entirely possible to thrive on a vegan diet, and many top athletes compete and win at the highest stages, while following a vegan diet. There are a whole host of other health benefits that you will see as a side effect of eating more plants, too, as well as being confident in the knowledge that you are living a more sustainable ethical life.

Being vegan is a privilege and not something that is available to everyone.
It's fair to say that eating well can be a privilege, mainly in terms of time and money. But that is true regardless of whether you are eating meat or not. Vegetables are generally cheaper than meat, especially if you are buying free-range meat. And if you are getting all your nutrients from low-budget, meat-focused prepared meals, then you'd better believe you'd be better off spending that money on colorful, market-bought veg.

What happens if I accidentally eat something that contains an animal product?
Don't worry about it! You're not going to be expelled from the vegan community for the occasional slipup. Any efforts you make toward a more plant-based life are going to have a positive impact on you and the planet, so give yourself a break and know what a brilliant thing you're doing for yourself and future generations.

Veganism is a fad. It may be popular right now, but sooner or later it'll be something else.
We don't agree. We see it more as a movement and a shift in behavior. The move away from smoking is something

that we don't believe will reverse as it was based on solid facts. The rise of vegan eating is based on similarly solid justifications about its benefits for the environment, our health, and animal welfare. Living vegan will grow until it's commonplace, and then the majority, and then onwards...

Veganism isn't going to solve the world's problems overnight. It's not going to solve world hunger and it's not going to solve climate change.
Correct, it's not going to solve all the world's problems overnight. The world is a very big place, and feeding its population is a hugely complicated issue. We need to consider soil health, seasonality of ingredients, and locality alongside many other issues. However, it's a big step in the right direction. Plant-based food is SO much more sustainable than animal products, and switching to a vegan diet would massively reduce our carbon footprint.

I've seen a photo of Ian wearing a leather belt and read your section on him wearing a leather jacket in the past, so therefore he's a hypocrite.
We've been on a journey, too! And it's taken a while for us to get to where we are today. Now, we don't tend to buy any new products that contain animals, but we can't be sure 100% of the time—no one can. Decisions we've made in the past have brought us to where we are now. We've come a long way, but we're also still learning all the time.

RESOURCES

Films

1. *Cowspiracy*
2. *Climate Change—The Facts*
3. *Earthlings*
4. *What the Health*
5. *The Most Important Speech You Will Ever Hear—* Gary Yourofsky
6. *Carnage*
7. *Okja*
8. *Food, Inc.*
9. *Forks Over Knives*
10. *Unity*

Books

1. *The Uninhabitable Earth—* David Wallace-Wells
2. *The China Study—* T. Colin Campbell
3. *Eating Animals—*Jonathan Safran Foer
4. *How Not to Die—* Dr. Michael Greger
5. *How to Create a Vegan World—*Tobias Leenaert
6. *No One is Too Small to Make a Difference—* Greta Thunberg
7. *30 Nonvegan Excuses & How to Respond to Them* (e-book)—Earthling Ed
8. *Why We Love Dogs, Eats Pigs, and Wear Cows—* Melanie Joy
9. *The Reducetarian Solution—* Brian Kateman
10. *Farmageddon—* Philip Lymbery

Online resources

1. www.vegansociety.com

2. www.peta.org

3. Plant Based News—
Instagram

4. **BOSH!**—all social channels

5. veganuary.com

6. vegnews.com

7. www.vegan.com

8. www.vivekindly.com

9. www.veganfoodandliving.
com

10. Joe Rogan Podcast #1259
In conversation with David
Wallace-Wells

Cookbook inspiration

1. **BOSH!** & **BISH BASH BOSH!**

2. Anna Jones:
   A Modern Way to Cook
   A Modern Way to Eat
   The Modern Cook's Year
   Many of these veggie recipes
   have vegan suggestions.

3. *The Wicked Healthy
   Cookbook*—Chad &
   Derek Sarno

4. *Vegan 100*—Gaz Oakley

5. *Vegan One Pound Meals*—
   Miguel Barclay

6. *Feed Me Vegan*—
   Lucy Watson

7. *What Vegans Eat*—
   Brett Cobley

8. *Veganomicon*—
   Isa Maskowitz &
   Terry Romero

9. *Thug Kitchen*

10. *So Vegan in 5*—Ben Park
    and Roxy Pope

Great food video channels and websites

1. BOSH.TV—Of course!

2. **Hot For Food**
Lauren Toyota is super personable and creates delicious dishes to please everyone.

3. **Avant-Garde Vegan**
Gaz's YouTube vids are beaut, complete with plants, pristine food, and beard styling.

4. **The Happy Pear**
The lads from Greystones are brimming with fun for life, healthy recipes, and how-to videos.

5. **Veganuary**

6. **Forks Over Knives**
These guys make incredibly healthy whole foods plant-based recipes, which look great.

7. **The Minimalist Baker**
A great source of baking inspiration, this blog is filled with simple dairy-free baking ideas.

8. **Vegan Richa**
If you're after authentic curries, then look no further than Vegan Richa's spicy creations.

9. **Deliciously Ella**
One of the first to popularize veggies, Ella makes plants cool again, and healthy, too.

10. **Jamie Oliver**
The big man himself is putting out more and more tasty plant-based recipes.

THANK-YOUS

Henry
Thanks to my family, friends, and everyone who experienced longer-than-acceptable response times on WhatsApp. Writing this book has been a mammoth task. Thanks to Ian for being a lifelong friend, for his culinary magic, and for holding the fort while I was holed up writing. Thanks to EmJ for putting your own world-changing business on hold for a moment to write part of this important book with us.

Ian
Thanks to my family, friends, and those people who surround me. Thanks for bearing with our madness and allowing me the freedom to build the life I choose. Thanks to Henry for his fierce hustle, his creativity, and for pulling himself away from the day-to-day to focus on cranking out the bulk of this important book, and Cathy and Charly for helping us spread delicious food and inspiration all over the world.

From both of us
Thanks to everyone who follows us and cooks our recipes, and all those we work with on a daily basis. Thanks to Lisa and every superstar at HarperCollins; Bev and Sarah at Bev James Management; Megan, Sarah, and all the team at Carver PR; Cassie and everyone at William Morrow; Dr. Alan Desmond, Dawn Carr, and Clare Gray for reading; and every single other person who has helped us on this journey. Let's all eat more plants!

REFERENCES

1 Ipsos Mori survey, commissioned by The Vegan Society, 2018, and The Food & You surveys, organised by the Food Standards Agency (FSA) and the National Centre for Social Science Research (Natcen).

2 Chiorando, M. (24 Jan. 2019). 93% of people buying vegan beyond meat products are also buying meat says report. Retrieved from https://www.plantbasednews.org/post/93-people-buying-vegan-beyond-meat-products-buying-meat.

3 Ipsos Mori survey, commissioned by The Vegan Society, 2018, and The Food & You surveys, organised by the Food Standards Agency (FSA) and the National Centre for Social Science Research (Natcen).

4 Carrington, D. (10 Jul. 2017). Earth's sixth mass extinction event under way, scientists warn. Retrieved from https://www.theguardian.com/environment/2017/jul/10/earths-sixth-mass-extinction-event-already-underway-scientists-warn.

5 Carrington, D. (30 Sep. 2014). Earth has lost half of its wildlife in the past 40 years, says WWF. Retrieved from https://www.theguardian.com/environment/2014/sep/29/earth-lost-50-wildlife-in-40-years-wwf.

6 Carrington, D. (21 May 2018). Humans just 0.01% of all life but have destroyed 83% of wild mammals—study. Retrieved from https://www.theguardian.com/environment/2018/may/21/human-race-just-001-of-all-life-but-has-destroyed-over-80-of-wild-mammals-study.

7 Carrington, D. (30 Sep. 2014). Earth has lost half of its wildlife in the past 40 years, says WWF. Retrieved from https://www.theguardian.com/environment/2014/sep/29/earth-lost-50-wildlife-in-40-years-wwf.

8 GSA Today (December 2012). Land transformation by humans: A review. Retrieved from http://www.geosociety.org/gsatoday/archive/22/12/abstract/i1052-5173-22-12-4.htm.

9 Bland, A. (1 Aug. 2012). Is the livestock industry destroying the planet? Retrieved from https://www.smithsonianmag.com/travel/is-the-livestock-industry-destroying-theplanet-11308007/.

10 Roberts, D. (19 Jan. 2018). This graphic explains why 2 degrees of global warming will be way worse than 1.5. Retrieved from https://www.vox.com/energy-and-environment/2018/1/19/16908402/global-warming-2-degrees-climate-change.

11 Illing, S. (24 Feb. 2019). It is absolutely time to panic about climate change. Retrieved from https://www.vox.com/energy-and-environment/2019/2/22/18188562/climate-change-david-wallace-wells-the-uninhabitable-earth.

12 France24 (13 Oct. 2018). Climate-related disasters increasing as temperatures rise, NGOs warn. Retrieved from https://www.france24.com/en/20181013-warn-more-climate-disasters-store-planet-warms-temperature.

13 NASA. Global climate change: Vital signs of the planet. Retrieved from https://climate.nasa.gov/.

14 Hsiang, S. M., Burke, M., and Miguel, E. (2013). Quantifying the influence of climate on human conflict. Science, 341(6151), 1235367. Retrieved from https://science.sciencemag.org/content/341/6151/1235367.

15 Union of Concerned Scientists. Causes of drought: What's the climate connection? Retrieved from https://www.ucsusa.org/global-warming/science-and-impacts/impacts/causes-of-drought-climate-change-connection.html.

16 Parker, L. (12 Jul. 2017). Sea level rise will flood hundreds of cities in the near future. Retrieved from https://news.nationalgeographic.com/2017/07/sea-level-rise-flood-global-warming-science/.

17 The World Bank (19 Mar. 2018). Groundswell: Preparing for internal climate migration [infographic]. Retrieved from https://www.worldbank.org/en/news/infographic/2018/03/19/groundswell---preparing-for-internal-climate-migration.

18 Phys.org (30 May 2018). Climate change hits poorest hardest, new research shows. Retrieved from https://phys.org/news/2018-05-climate-poorest-hardest.html.

19 Wikipedia. Environmental migrant. Retrieved from https://en.wikipedia.org/wiki/Environmental_migrant.

20 World Food Programme (15 Sep. 2017). World hunger again on the rise, driven by conflict and climate change, new UN report says. Retrieved from https://www1.wfp.org/news/world-hunger-again-rise-driven-conflict-and-climate-change-new-un-report-says.

21 Illing, S. (24 Feb. 2019). It is absolutely time to panic about climate change. Retrieved from https://www.vox.com/energy-and-environment/2019/2/22/18188562/climate-change-david-wallace-wells-the-uninhabitable-earth.

22 Revkin, A. (July 2018). Climate change first became news 30 years ago. Why haven't we fixed it? Retrieved from https://www.nationalgeographic.com/magazine/2018/07/embark-essay-climate-change-pollution-revkin/.

23 Turrentine, J. (12 Oct. 2018). Climate scientists to world: We have only 20 years before there's no turning back. Retrieved from https://www.nrdc.org/onearth/climate-scientists-world-we-have-only-20-years-theres-no-turning-back.

24 Carrington, D. (26 Apr. 2019). "Outrage is justified": David Attenborough backs school climate strikers. Retrieved from https://www.theguardian.com/environment/2019/apr/26/david-attenborough-backs-school-climate-strikes-outrage-greta-thunberg.

25 Waterman, C. (22 Apr. 2019). The High Cost of Cheap Meat. Retrieved from https://fairworldproject.org/the-high-cost-of-cheap-meat/.

26 Davies, M., Wasley, A., (17 July 2017). Intensive Farming in the UK, by Numbers. Retrieved from https://www.thebureauinvestigates.com/stories/2017-07-17/intensive-numbers-of-intensive-farming.

27 Human Research Council (Dec. 2014). Study of current and former vegetarians and vegans. Retrieved from https://faunalytics.org/wp-content/uploads/2015/06/Faunalytics_Current-Former-Vegetarians_Full-Report.pdf.

28 Turner-McGrievy, G. M., Barnard, N. D., and Scialli, A. R. (2007). A two-year randomized weight loss trial comparing a vegan diet to a more moderate low-fat diet. Obesity, 15(9), 2276–2281. Retrieved from https://www.ncbi.nlm.nih.gov/pubmed/17890496.

29 Tonstad, S., Butler, T., Yan, R., and Fraser, G. E. (2009). Type of vegetarian diet, body weight, and prevalence of type 2 diabetes.

Diabetes Care, 32(5), 791–796. Retrieved from https://www.ncbi.nlm.nih.gov/pubmed/19351712.

30 Diabetes UK. Vegetarian diets and diabetes. Retrieved from https://www.diabetes.org.uk/guide-to-diabetes/enjoy-food/eating-with-diabetes/vegetarian-diets.

31 Kahleova H., Levin, S., Barnard, N. (June 2018). Vegetarian Dietary Patterns and Cardiovascular Disease. Retrieved from https://www.sciencedirect.com/science/article/abs/pii/S0033062018300872

32 Nuccitelli, D. (15 Oct. 2018). There's one key takeaway from last week's IPCC report. Retrieved from https://www.theguardian.com/environment/climate-consensus-97-per-cent/2018/oct/15/theres-one-key-takeaway-from-last-weeks-ipcc-report.

33 Khan, A. (3 Nov. 2016). How much Arctic sea ice are you melting? Scientists have an answer. Retrieved from https://www.latimes.com/science/sciencenow/la-sci-sn-co2-sea-ice-20161103-story.html.

34 Petter, O. (1 Jun. 2018). Veganism is "single biggest way" to reduce our environmental impact on planet, study finds. Retrieved from https://www.independent.co.uk/life-style/health-and-families/veganism-environmental-impact-planetreduced-plant-based-diet-humansstudy-a8378631.html.

35 Hill, T. (3 May 2019). Dropping red meat from one meal a week could slash emissions eight per cent, study shows. Retrieved from https://www.businessgreen.com/bg/news-analysis/3074895/dropred-meat-from-one-meal-per-week-toslash-emissions-by-8-per-cent-studysays.

36 The Humane Society of the United States. Meatless Mondays Toolkit for Parents. Retrieved from https://www.humanesociety.org/sites/default/files/docs/meatless-mondays-toolkit-parents.pdf

37 Oppenlander, R. (20 Aug. 2013). Animal agriculture, hunger, and how to feed a growing global population: Part one of two. Retrieved from https://www.forksoverknives.com/animal-agriculture-hunger-and-how-to-feed-a-growing-global-population-part-one-of-two.

38 Million Dollar Vegan. World hunger. Retrieved from https://www.milliondollarvegan.com/en-au/why/world-hunger/.

39 Carrington, D. (31 May 2018). Avoiding meat and dairy is "single biggest way" to reduce your impact on Earth. Retrieved from https://www.theguardian.com/environment/2018/may/31/avoiding-meat-and-dairy-is-single-biggest-way-to-reduce-your-impact-on-earth.

40 University of Oxford (22 Mar. 2016). Veggie-based diets could save 8 million lives by 2050 and cut global warming. Retrieved from http://www.ox.ac.uk/news/2016-03-22-veggie-based-diets-could-save-8-million-lives-2050-and-cut-global-warming.

41 Scientific American. How does meat in the diet take an environmental toll? Retrieved from https://www.scientificamerican.com/article/meat-and-environment/.

42 Poore, J., Nemeck, T., (1 Jun. 2018). Reducing food's environmental impacts through producers and consumers. Retrieved from https://josephpoore.com/Science%20360%206392%20987%20-%20Accepted%20Manuscript.pdf.

43 Whyte, C. (20 Sept. 2018). Milk alternatives: Which are good for both you and the planet? Retrieved from http://liliec.be/resume/Heath-Food/Milk%20alternatives

%20Which%20are%20good%20for%20
both%20you%20and%20the%20planet.pdf

44 Poore, J., and Nemecek, T. (2018).
Reducing food's environmental impacts
through producers and consumers.
Science, 360(6392), 987–992. Retrieved
from https://science.sciencemag.org/
content/360/6392/987.

45 Shepon, A., Eshel, G., Noor, E., and
Milo, R. (2016). Energy and protein
feed-to-food conversion efficiencies in
the US and potential food security gains
from dietary changes. Environmental
Research Letters, 11(10), 105002.
Retrieved from https://iopscience.iop.org/
article/10.1088/1748-9326/11/10/105002.

46 Mekonnen, M. M., and Hoekstra, A. Y.
(2010). The green, blue and grey water
footprint of farm animals and animal
products (Vol. 1). UNESCO-IHE. Retrieved
from https://waterfootprint.org/media/
downloads/Report-48-WaterFootprint-
AnimalProducts-Vol1.pdf.

47 Hoekstra, A. Y., and Mekonnen, M. M.
(2012). The water footprint of humanity.
Proceedings of the National Academy of
Sciences, 109(9), 3232–3237. Retrieved
from https://www.ncbi.nlm.nih.gov/
pubmed/22331890.

48 Million Dollar Vegan (10 Feb. 2019).
The impact of meat and dairy on the
planet—Dr Joseph Poore (Part 1) [video].
Retrieved from https://www.youtube.com/
watch?v=qLkqkyTMLlw.

49 Ibid.

50 Monbiot, G. (3 Apr. 2019). The natural
world can help save us from climate
catastrophe. Retrieved from https://www.
theguardian.com/commentisfree/2019/
apr/03/natural-world-climate-catastrophe-
rewilding.

51 Viegas, J. (16 Sep. 2015). Half of all marine
life lost in 40 years: WWF report. Retrieved
from https://www.abc.net.au/news/
science/2015-09-16/half-marine-life-lostin-
40-years/6779912.

52 Fujita, R. (11 Jul. 2012). FAO reports 87%
of the world's fisheries are overexploited
or fully exploited [blog]. Retrieved from
http://blogs.edf.org/edfish/2012/07/11/fao-
reports-87-of-the-worlds-fisheries-are-
overexploited-or-fully-exploited/.

53 Myers, R. A., and Worm, B. (2005).
Extinction, survival or recovery of large
predatory fishes. Philosophical Transactions
of the Royal Society B: Biological Sciences,
360(1453), 13–20. Retrieved from https://
www.ncbi.nlm.nih.gov/pmc/articles/
PMC1636106/.

54 CBS News (2 Nov. 2006). Salt-water fish
extinction seen by 2048. Retrieved from
https://www.cbsnews.com/news/salt-
water-fish-extinction-seen-by-2048/.

55 Viegas, J. (16 Sep. 2015). Half of all
marine life lost in 40 years: WWF report.
Retrieved from https://www.abc.net.au/
news/science/2015-09-16/half-marine-life-
lostin-40-years/6779912.

56 Food and Agriculture Organization of
the United Nations. Discards and bycatch in
Shrimp trawl fisheries. Retrieved from http://
www.fao.org/3/W6602E/w6602E09.htm.

57 Food and Agriculture Organization of the
United Nations (13 Oct. 2009). How to feed
the world in 2050. Retrieved from http://
www.fao.org/fileadmin/templates/wsfs/
docs/expert_paper/How_to_Feed_the_
World_in_2050.pdf.

58 Oppenlander, R. (26 Aug. 2013). Animal
agriculture, hunger, and how to feed a
growing global population: Part two of two.
Retrieved from https://www.forksoverknives.

com/animal-agriculture-hunger-and-how-to-feed-a-growing-global-population-part-two-of-two/.

59 The Conversation (26 Apr. 2017). Five ways the meat on your plate is killing the planet. Retrieved from http://theconversation.com/five-ways-the-meat-on-your-plate-is-killing-the-planet-76128.

60 Million Dollar Vegan (10 Feb. 2019). The impact of meat and dairy on the planet—Dr Joseph Poore (Part 1) [video]. Retrieved from https://www.youtube.com/watch?v=qLkqkyTMLlw.

61 Good, K. Explain like I'm 5: Why tofu consumption is not responsible for soy-related deforestation. Retrieved from https://www.onegreenplanet.org/environment/why-tofu-consumption-is-not-responsible-for-soy-related-deforestation/.

62 Taylor, M. (18 Jul. 2018). Is soy good or bad for you? Here's the science-backed answer. Retrieved from https://www.goodhousekeeping.com/health/dietnutrition/a20707020/is-soy-good-or-bad-for-you/.

63 Global Forest Atlas. Soy Agriculture in the Amazon Basin. Retrieved from https://globalforestatlas.yale.edu/amazon/land-use/soy.

64 COWSPIRACY. The facts. Retrieved from http://www.cowspiracy.com/facts.

65 Good, K. Explain like I'm 5: Why tofu consumption is not responsible for soy-related deforestation. Retrieved from https://www.onegreenplanet.org/environment/why-tofu-consumption-is-not-responsible-for-soy-related-deforestation/.

66 Khan Academy. The United Nations. Retrieved from https://www.khanacademy.org/humanities/us-history/rise-to-world-power/us-wwii/a/the-united-nations.

67 Rich, N. (1 Aug. 2018). Losing Earth: The decade we almost stopped climate change. Retrieved from https://www.nytimes.com/interactive/2018/08/01/magazine/climate-change-losing-earth.html.

68 Physicians Committee for Responsible Medicine. Lowering cholesterol with a plant-based diet. Retrieved from https://www.pcrm.org/good-nutrition/nutrition-information/lowering-cholesterol-with-a-plant-based-diet.

69 Diabetes UK. Vegetarian diets and diabetes. Retrieved from https://www.diabetes.org.uk/guide-to-diabetes/enjoy-food/eating-with-diabetes/vegetarian-diets.

70 University of Oxford (12 Oct. 2018). Balanced plant-based diets improve our health and the health of the planet. Retrieved from http://www.ox.ac.uk/news/2018-10-12-balanced-plant-based-diets-improve-our-health-and-health-planet.

71 vegsource.com (16 May 2010). World Health Org and UN recommend populations eat plant-based diets. Retrieved from http://www.vegsource.com/news/2010/05/world-health-org-and-un-recommend-populations-eat-plant-based-diets.html.

72 Tello, M. (29 Nov. 2018). Eat more plants, fewer animals [blog]. Retrieved from https://www.health.harvard.edu/blog/eat-more-plants-fewer-animals-2018112915198.

73 Harvard Health Publishing (1 Jan. 2018). The right plant-based diet for you. Retrieved from https://www.health.harvard.edu/staying-healthy/the-right-plant-based-diet-for-you.

74 University of Oxford (12 Oct. 2018). Balanced plant-based diets improve our health and the health of the planet. Retrieved from http://www.ox.ac.uk/news/2018-10-12-balanced-plant-based-diets-improve-our-health-and-health-planet.

75 Government of Canada (2 Apr. 2019). Canada's food guide. Retrieved from https://food-guide.canada.ca/en/.

76 Physicians Committee for Responsible Medicine (3 Mar. 2016). Processed meat and fish increase risk for breast cancer. Retrieved from https://www.pcrm.org/news/health-nutrition/processed-meat-and-fish-increase-risk-breast-cancer.

77 Press Association (12 Mar. 2012). Eating red meat raises "substantially" risk of cancer or heart disease death. Retrieved from https://www.theguardian.com/science/2012/mar/12/red-meat-death-heart-cancer.

78 Tuso, P., Stoll, S. R., and Li, W. W. (2015). A plant-based diet, atherogenesis, and coronary artery disease prevention. The Permanente Journal, 19(1), 62. Retrieved from https://www.ncbi.nlm.nih.gov/pubmed/25431999.

79 World Health Organization (Oct. 2015). Q&A on the carcinogenicity of the consumption of red meat and processed meat. Retrieved from https://www.who.int/features/qa/cancer-red-meat/en/.

80 US Food & Drug Administration (31 Mar. 2004). FDA/EPA 2004 Advice on what you need to know about mercury in fish and shellfish. Retrieved from https://www.fda.gov/food/metals/what-you-need-know-about-mercury-fish-and-shellfish.

81 NHS Inform (9 Jul. 2019). Food poisoning. Retrieved from https://www.nhsinform.scot/illnesses-and-conditions/infections-and-poisoning/food-poisoning.

82 Viva! Health. Food poisoning. Retrieved from https://www.vivahealth.org.uk/resources/meat-truth/food-poisoning-online.

83 Mosley, M. (21 Feb. 2018). The dirtiest place in your kitchen might surprise you . . . Retrieved from https://www.bbc.co.uk/news/health-43131764.

84 Poppick, S. (8 Oct. 2015). Here's how much money vegetarians save each year. Retrieved from http://money.com/money/4066188/vegetarians-save-money/.

85 Annemans, L. (14 Feb. 2018). Plant-based eating is cost-effective. Retrieved from http://www.alprofoundation.org/news-events/plant-based-eating-is-cost-effective/.

86 Robson, D. (18 Jan. 2019). A high-carb diet may explain why Okinawans live so long. Retrieved from http://www.bbc.com/future/story/20190116-a-high-carb-diet-may-explain-why-okinawans-live-so-long.

87 Sobiecki, J. G., Appleby, P. N., Bradbury, K. E., and Key, T. J. (2016). High compliance with dietary recommendations in a cohort of meat eaters, fish eaters, vegetarians, and vegans: results from the European Prospective Investigation into Cancer and Nutrition—Oxford study. Nutrition Research, 36(5), 464–477. doi:10.1016/j.nutres.2015.12.016.

88 American Dietetic Association. Position of the American Dietetic Association: Vegetarian Diets. Journal of the Academy of Nutrition and Dietetics, 2009; 109 (7): 1266-1282 DOI: 10.1016/j.jada.2009.05.027.

89 The Association of UK Dieticians. (7 Aug. 2017). British Dietetic Association confirms well-planned vegan diets can support healthy living in people of all ages. Retrieved from https://www.bda.uk.com/news/view?id=179.

90 Tucker, K. L., Rich, S., Rosenberg, I., Jacques, P., Dallal, G., Wilson, P. W., and Selhub, J. (2000). Plasma vitamin B-12

concentrations relate to intake source in the Framingham Offspring study. The American Journal of Clinical Nutrition, 71(2), 514–522. Retrieved from https://www.ncbi.nlm.nih.gov/pubmed/10648266.

91 Craig, W. J. (2009). Health effects of vegan diets. The American Journal of Clinical Nutrition, 89(5), 1627S–1633S. Retrieved from https://academic.oup.com/ajcn/article/89/5/1627S/4596952.

92 Matthews-King, A. (4 Apr. 2019). Western diet now killing more than smoking and high blood pressure, study suggests. Retrieved from https://www.independent.co.uk/news/health/Western-diet-fat-salt-fruit-veg-fiber-cancer-heart-disease-obesity-diabetes-a8853696.html.

93 Downer, M. K., Martínez-González, M. A., Gea, A., Stampfer, M., Warnberg, J., Ruiz-Canela, M., . . . and Estruch, R. (2017). Mercury exposure and risk of cardiovascular disease: a nested case-control study in the PREDIMED (PREvention with MEDiterranean Diet) study. BMC Cardiovascular Disorders, 17(1), 9. Retrieved from https://www.ncbi.nlm.nih.gov/pmc/articles/PMC5216562/.

94 Smithers, R. (1 Nov. 2018). Third of Britons have stopped or reduced eating meat—report. Retrieved from https://www.theguardian.com/business/2018/nov/01/third-of-britons-have-stopped-or-reduced-meat-eating-vegan-vegetarian-report.

95 Chiorando, M. (27 Mar. 2019). "93% of flexitarians won't go vegan within 12 months" says YouGov report. Retrieved from https://www.plantbasednews.org/post/most-flexitarians-wont-go-vegan-12-months.

96 Forgrieve, J. (2 Nov. 2018). The growing acceptance of veganism. Retrieved from https://www.forbes.com/sites/janetforgrieve/2018/11/02/picturing-a-kindler-gentler-world-vegan-month/.

97 Wohl, J. (1 Apr. 2019). How the rise of "flexitarians" is powering plant-based foods. Retrieved from https://adage.com/article/cmo-strategy/power-plant-based-food/317167.

98 Terazano, E. (23 Dec. 2018). Oat milk sales surge as more consumers go dairy-free. Retrieved from https://www.ft.com/content/4824217e-0527-11e9-99df-6183d3002ee1.

99 Murphy, M. (5 May 2019). Beyond Meat soars 163% in biggest-popping U.S. IPO since 2000. Retrieved from https://www.marketwatch.com/story/beyond-meat-soars-163-in-biggest-popping-us-ipo-since-2000-2019-05-02.

100 Shashwat, A., Muvija, M. (14 May 2019). Vegan sausage rolls rake in the dough for Greggs, shares hit record. Retrieved from https://uk.reuters.com/article/uk-greggs-outlook/vegan-sausage-rolls-rake-in-the-dough-for-greggs-shares-hit-record-idUKKCN1SK0OD.

101 Ashworth, W. (4 Oct. 2018). 7 stocks to buy to ride the vegan wave. Retrieved from https://investorplace.com/2018/10/7-stocks-to-buy-to-ride-the-vegan-wave/.

102 VegFAQs (28 May 2019). Best vegan companies to invest in: public and private stock options. Retrieved from https://vegfaqs.com/vegan-companies-to-invest-in/.

103 Chiorando, M. (9 Oct 2018). 'Avocados And Butternut Squash Are Not Vegan' Claims BBC Show QI. Retrieved from https://www.plantbasednews.org/post/avocados-butternut-squash-not-vegan-bbc-qi.

104 Winch, S. Hot topic: Is palm oil vegan [blog]. Retrieved from https://veganuary.com/blog/hot-topic-is-palm-oil-vegan/.

105 Veganuary. Vegan label reading guide. Retrieved from https://veganuary.com/starter-kit/vegan-label-reading-guide/.

106 Veganuary. Vegan label reading guide: E numbers. Retrieved from https://veganuary.com/starter-kit/vegan-label-reading-guide/e-numbers/.

107 Eat By Date. How long do beans last? Retrieved from https://www.eatbydate.com/proteins/beans-peas/beans-shelf-life-expiration-date/.

108 Guibourg, C. and Briggs, H. (22 Feb. 2019). Climate change: Which vegan milk is best? Retrieved from https://www.bbc.co.uk/news/science-environment-46654042.

109 Ibid.

110 McDougall, A. (20 Aug. 2018). How can beauty companies make the most of veganism's rising popularity? Retrieved from https://www.mintel.com/blog/beauty-market-news/how-can-beauty-companies-make-the-most-of-veganisms-rising-popularity.

111 The Tasty Vegan. Nonvegan makeup ingredients. Retrieved from http://www.thetastyvegan.com/vegan-shopping/vegan-cosmetics-and-toiletries/vegan-makeup/nonvegan-makeup-ingredients/.

112 Peters, J. (29 Jun. 2019). "Is there such a thing as vegan loo roll?": How to have a cruelty-free home. Retrieved from https://www.theguardian.com/lifeandstyle/2019/jun/29/is-there-such-a-thing-as-vegan-loo-roll-how-to-have-a-cruelty-free-home.

113 Ibid.

114 Galliers, L. (19 Oct. 2011). Where will your coffee cup end up? Not in the recycling. Retrieved from https://conversation.which.co.uk/fooddrink/recycling-disposable-coffee-cups-starbucks/.

115 Parliament UK (22 Dec. 2017). Coffee cup waste in the UK. Retrieved from https://publications.parliament.uk/pa/cm201719/cmselect/cmenvaud/657/65705.htm#footnote-078-backlink.

116 Loria, J. (29 Jun. 2018). Straws aren't the real problem. Fishing nets account for 46 percent of all ocean plastic. Retrieved from https://mercyforanimals.org/straws-arent-the-real-problem-fishing-nets.

117 Parker, L. (22 Mar. 2018). The Great Pacific Garbage Patch isn't what you think it is. Retrieved from https://news.nationalgeographic.com/2018/03/great-pacific-garbage-patch-plastics-environment/.

118 Elsey, W. (30 May 2018). Why your company should be more socially responsible. Retrieved from https://www.forbes.com/sites/.

119 Carrington, D. (31 May 2018). Avoiding meat and dairy is "single biggest way" to reduce your impact on Earth. Retrieved from https://www.theguardian.com/environment/2018/may/31/avoiding-meat-and-dairy-is-single-biggest-way-to-reduce-your-impact-on-earth.businessdevelopmentcouncil/2018/05/30/why-your-company-should-be-more-socially-responsible/.

BOSH!: HOW TO LIVE VEGAN. Copyright © 2019 by Henry Firth and Ian Theasby. All rights reserved. Printed in the United States of America. No part of this book may be used or reproduced in any manner whatsoever without written permission except in the case of brief quotations embodied in critical articles and reviews. For information, address HarperCollins Publishers, 195 Broadway, New York, NY 10007.

HarperCollins books may be purchased for educational, business, or sales promotional use. For information, please email the Special Markets Department at SPsales@harpercollins.com.

Originally published in Great Britain in 2019 by HQ, an imprint of HarperCollinsPublishers Ltd. 2019.

FIRST U.S. EDITION

Project editor and Researcher: Laura Herring
Page design: Louise Evans
Illustration: Martha and Hepsie (marthaandhepsie.com)
Vegan Make-Up Expert: Em-J (@emj.makeupartist)

Library of Congress Cataloging-in-Publication Data has been applied for.

ISBN 978-0-06-296990-3

19 20 21 22 23   DIX/LSC   10 9 8 7 6 5 4 3 2 1